Aids to Medicine for Dental

Aids to Medicine for Dental Students

R. W. Matthews
PhD MDS BDS
Lecturer in Oral Medicine, University of Bristol

J. L. Burton
BSc MD FRCP
Consultant and Senior Lecturer in Dermatology, University of
Bristol

CHURCHILL LIVINGSTONE
EDINBURGH LONDON MELBOURNE AND NEW YORK 1983

CHURCHILL LIVINGSTONE
Medical Division of Longman Group Limited

Distributed in the United States of America by
Churchill Livingstone Inc., 1560 Broadway, New
York, N.Y. 10036, and by associated companies,
branches and representatives throughout the
world.

First published 1983

ISBN 0 443 02690 4

British Library Cataloguing in Publication Data
Matthews, R. W.
    Aids to medicine for dental students.
    1. Medicine   2. Dentistry
    I. Title   II. Burton, J. L.
    610' .246176   RT65

Library of Congress Cataloging in Publication Data
Matthews, R. W.
    Aids to medicine for dental students.
    Includes index.
    1. Internal medicine.   2. Dental students.
I. Burton, J. L. (John Lloyd)   II. Title.
[DNLM: 1. Medicine. WB 100 M441a]
RC46.M43   1983   616' .00246176
82-23452

Printed in Singapore
by The Print House Pte Ltd

Preface

This little book gives a concise summary of selected topics in general medicine.

It is hoped that the information will be useful to dental undergraduates, postgraduates and established dental practitioners. Thus the amount of detail included has been made sufficiently extensive to cover these varying needs. Obviously, many medical topics have been omitted, as they were not thought relevant. Time will tell whether our selection was right. Suggestions or comments for improvement will be welcomed.

It has been assumed that the reader has a basic knowledge of medicine. Reference to more extensive textbooks may be necessary to explain terms or conditions listed in the book with which the reader is not familiar.

Dentists have regular contact with their patients, unlike most medical practitioners who are consulted only when a patient is ill. The dentist has a heavy responsibility to recognise those of his patients who require referral to a medical practitioner. He also has a responsibility to consult a patient's physician when dental treatment is complicated by the medical condition of the patient. Both these responsibilities require that the dentist has adequate medical training. It is hoped that this book will provide a useful and quick method to obtain medical information relevant to the practice of dentistry.

Bristol 1983   R.W.M.
                                                                   J.L.B.

Contents

Contents

Cardiovascular system

THE PULSE

Arterial
Usually palpated in radial artery at the wrist. Can also be felt in the carotid, subclavian, facial and brachial arteries. Arterial pulses in legs may also provide useful information, e.g. diminished by atheroma, delayed by aortic coarctation.

Characteristics
1. Rate — normally 60–90 beats per minute at rest
2. Rhythm — regular or irregular
3. Volume — weak ('thready'), normal or increased volume ('bounding')
4. Rigidity of wall — often increased in older subjects, but poor correlation with arterial disease.

Venous
Best seen in jugular veins.

Jugular venous pressure (JVP)
With the patient resting at 30° to horizontal, the jugular veins should not be filled to a vertical height of 4 cm above the sternal angle. Elevated JVP is an important sign.

Causes of raised JVP
1. Hyperdynamic circulation
    (i) Exercise
   (ii) Fever
  (iii) Anaemia
  (iv) Thyrotoxicosis
   (v) Pregnancy
  (vi) AV fistulae
2. Right ventricular failure
3. Obstruction of superior vena cava
4. Tricuspid stenosis or incompetence
5. Pericardial effusion

6. Fluid overload (especially i.v. infusion)
7. Very slow heart rate

HEART SOUNDS

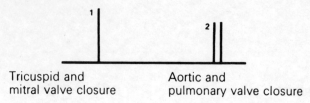

Tricuspid and   Aortic and
mitral valve closure   pulmonary valve closure

Fig. 1 Heart sounds.
(Reproduced from Burton J L 1980 Aids to undergraduate medicine, 3rd
edn, with permission.)

1. Aortic valve normally closes before pulmonary valve.
2. Pulmonary closure is delayed by inspiration (due to increased
   venous return caused by decreased intrathoracic pressure). The
   normal split therefore widens on inspiration.

First sound
Loud in
1. Mitral stenosis
2. Hyperdynamic circulation
3. Tachycardia
Soft in
1. Mitral incompetence
2. Rheumatic carditis
3. Severe heart failure

Second sound in aortic area
Loud in systemic hypertension
Soft in aortic stenosis

Second sound in pulmonary area
Loud in pulmonary hypertension
Soft in pulmonary stenosis
A third heart sound and fourth heart sound are sometimes heard.
A third sound is frequently found in healthy young people but is
abnormal over the age of 40. A fourth heart sound (heard at the
lower end of the sternum) always indicates disease.
Note rate, rhythm and character of the sounds. Abnormal sounds
or murmurs may indicate serious disease and require expert
diagnosis. Obviously, such cases are unsuitable for general
anaesthesia in a dental surgery.

APEX BEAT

Heart is enlarged or displaced if apex beat is:
1. Lateral to midclavicular line
2. Below 5th intercostal space

Causes of absent apex beat
1. Obesity
2. Emphysema
3. Pericardial effusion
4. Shock
5. Dextrocardia

Disorders of heart rate and rhythm

TACHYCARDIA
Increased heart rate above normal. May be physiological (exercise, emotion) or pathological (fevers, esp. rheumatic fever, thyrotoxicosis and drugs, e.g. adrenaline).
Paroxysmal Tachycardia: Spontaneous increase in heart rate characterized by sudden onset and cessation.
Tachycardia may not lead to serious complications in the undamaged heart. Those with pre-existing heart disease may suffer cardiac failure as a result of the extra work involved in dealing with a sudden rapid heart rate.

Extrasystoles
Premature beats occurring out of time with the normal heart rhythm. Usually followed by *compensatory pause.* Often caused by excessive smoking or drinking. They are often of little significance but may be due to drugs, e.g. digitalis, or heart disease. Usually abolished by exercise.

Fibrillation
Unco-ordinated muscle twitching in the heart. Results in poor heart function.

Atrial fibrillation
Common disorder. Most frequently occurs in
1. Mitral stenosis
2. Thyrotoxicosis
3. Myocardial ischaemia
Ventricles beat irregularly as a result of atrial fibrillation — produces a rapid pulse which is irregular in time and volume.
Auricles do not contract, so blood clots and becomes attached to auricular wall. Fragments may break away and cause systemic embolism, resulting e.g. in a 'stroke'.

Ventricular fibrillation
produces ineffective cardiac contraction. Syncope (sudden loss of
consciousness due to cerebral hypoxia) is followed rapidly by
death.
Caused by
1. Myocardial ischaemia or infarction
2. Drugs e.g. Adrenaline injections or intravenous digoxin
3. May follow ventricular paroxysmal tachycardia.

Bradycardia
Slow heart rate. Common in myxoedema and raised intra-cranial
pressure. Profound bradycardia is produced in *Heart block* — a
block in the conduction mechanism in the heart from the
pacemaker (sino-atrial node) via the AV node to the Bundle of His
and the ventricular myocardium. In complete heart block the
ventricles beat at their own slow inherent rate as they lack stimuli
from the pacemaker. The rate may be as low as 40 beats a minute
or less. Such a low heart rate should always suggest complete
heart block. The condition occurs most often in elderly males with
ischaemic heart disease.

Stokes-Adams attack
This is a period of unconsciousness from cerebral anoxia due to
transient cardiac arrest as a result of unstable heart block. Expert
attention is required to manage this eventuality.

CARDIAC FAILURE

A state where the myocardium cannot maintain the normal
circulation. It is *not* cardiac arrest, though this does cause cardiac
failure.
Severity estimated by amount of exertion required to produce
breathlessness (dyspnoea).
Either the L. side or the R. side of the heart may fail first, but
eventually both sides will be involved.

Common causes of cardiac failure
1. Hypertension
2. Ischaemic heart disease
3. Valvular disease
4. Chronic pulmonary disease

Right ventricular failure (Congestive cardiac failure)
Increased venous pressure due to incomplete emptying of the right
side of the heart, which receives venous blood from the peripheral
circulation.

Causes
1. Following L. ventricular failure
2. Mitral stenosis
3. Cor pulmonale, secondary to pulmonary disease e.g. chronic bronchitis or pulmonary embolism.
4. Congenital heart disease

Symptoms
1. Tiredness, weakness
2. Oedema
3. GI upset, anorexia and may be hepatic pain (all due to venous engorgement of abdominal viscera)

Signs
1. Raised JVP — seen as conspicuous jugular veins in the neck of resting patient
2. Dependent oedema (ankles or sacral area)
3. Large tender liver
4. May be ascites and pleural effusion
5. Functional tricuspid incompetence due to stretching of the AV ring
6. Oliguria by day; nocturia. Concentrated urine with albuminuria is common
7. Peripheral cyanosis in severe cases

Left ventricular failure
Here the venous congestion is not readily seen as it is the pulmonary veins which are affected. Thus pulmonary effects predominate.

Causes
1. Myocardial ischaemia
2. Hypertension
3. Aortic stenosis or incompetence
4. Mitral incompetence

Symptoms
1. Exertional dyspnoea
2. Orthopnoea
3. Paroxysmal nocturnal dyspnoea, often with coughing and wheezing
4. Pulmonary oedema (anxiety, dyspnoea, cough and pink frothy sputum)

Signs
1. Tachycardia
2. Enlarged heart
3. Gallop rhythm

4. May be functional mitral incompetence due to stretched AV ring
5. Crackles at lung bases; may be rhonchi
6. Cheyne-Stokes breathing may occur in sedated elderly patients

Principles of treatment of cardiac failure
1. *Rest*
2. *Lowering venous pressre*
   (i) Digitalis therapy
   (ii) Diuretics (with potassium supplementation) orally
   (iii) Reduce salt intake
3. *Antihypertensive therapy* if hypertension is the cause of cardiac failure
4. Severe cases may need *oxygen therapy*, i.v. frusemide, etc

HYPERTENSION — persistently raised blood pressure

Normal B.P. (in mmHg) — *Systolic*: 100 plus age of patient
                         Diastolic: 60–85
High *diastolic* B.P. is the more serious; it causes arterial degeneration and places a stress on the myocardium.
Any patient with a B.P. of 160/100 must be considered to have hypertension.

Types of hypertension
1. *Primary* (essential). Cause unknown. 'Malignant' hypertension is a severe form characterized by retinal changes and progressive renal failure.
2. *Secondary* due to
   (i) Renal ischaemia (remember renin/angiotensin) or nephritis
   (ii) Rarely Cushings disease; phaeochromocytoma or aortic coarctation
   (iii) Toxaemia of pregnancy (may require termination of pregnancy)

Effects of hypertension
(A) *On the heart:*
    1. Myocardial hypertrophy
    2. Left ventricular failure

(B) On the arteries:
    Atheroma. This may cause:
    1. Coronary artery occlusion giving pain (angina pectoris) due to cardiac ischaemia or infarction
    2. Cerebral vascular insufficiency leading e.g. to senile dementia

3. Cerebral thrombosis or haemorrhage ('stroke') leading to loss of function of the affected part of brain, e.g. speech defects when Broca's area affected; contralateral hemiplegia when motor cortex affected
4. Visual disturbances due to retinal vessel damage and papilloedema
5. Renal artery occlusion leading to renal ischaemia, itself a cause of hypertension (renin/angiotensin)

Common symptoms of hypertension
1. Headache, giddiness, palpitations
2. Breathelessness
3. Angina of effort
4. Visual disturbances

Signs
1. Elevated systemic B.P. Full pulse, difficult to obliterate
2. Displacement of apex beat outwards and downwards, due to ventricular hypertrophy
3. Papilloedema and retinal haemorrhages or exudates
4. May be albuminuria if renal damage is present
5. May be signs of cardiac failure
   The most important complications and causes of death from hypertension are
1. Cardiac failure
2. Cerebral thrombosis or haemorrhage ('stroke')
3. Uraemia

Treatment of hypertension
1. Removal of cause if possible e.g. ischaemic kidney, phaeochromocytoma
2. Reduction of weight
3. Rest and diminution of stress (? tranquillizers)
4. Diuretics (with potassium supplementation)
5. Hypotensive drugs

VALVULAR HEART DISEASE
The main causes of valvular disease of the heart are
1. *Congenital defects.* May cause septal defects as well as valvular disease.
2. *Rheumatic fever.* Becoming rare in UK; commonly mitral and aortic valves affected.
Valvular heart disease causes disturbance of blood flow through the valves. This may change the characteristic heart sounds or produce extra sounds called *murmurs.* The vibrations of blood turbulence transmitted to the chest wall may be felt as *thrills.* The disturbed blood flow may cause heart failure.

Dental significance of valvular heart disease
These patients are more susceptible to bacterial endocarditis from a bacteraemia. Tooth removal, apicectomy and gingival surgery as well as subgingival scaling cause bleeding and an inevitable bacteraemia. Thus, these patients must receive prophylactic antibiotics prior to such procedures (antibiotic cover — p. 11).

TYPES OF VALVULAR DISEASE OF THE HEART

1. Mitral incompetence
This defect allows blood to re-enter the left atrium during ventricular contraction (systole) instead of the blood being entirely expelled into the aorta. The murmur caused by the forceful regurgitation of blood across the incompetent valve therefore occurs during systole.

2. Mitral stenosis
Emptying of the left atrium into the left ventricle is hampered by the restricted opening of the mitral valve. This causes hypertrophy of the left atrium as it tries to overcome the obstruction. The murmur produced by passage of blood across the damaged valve during atrial contraction occurs when the ventricle is in diastole — thus this murmur is heard during diastole.

3. Aortic incompetence
Left ventricular contraction expels blood into the aorta. As soon as the left ventricle relaxes (diastole) the elastic recoil of the aorta expels the blood back into the left ventricle if the valve is incompetent. Consequently the peripheral pulse has an unsustained character and is called a *collapsing pulse*. The blood regurgitation occurs during ventricular diastole and therefore produces a diastolic murmur.

4. Aortic stenosis
There is obstruction to blood flow from the left ventricle into the aorta during ventricular systole and the murmur produced is therefore systolic. Due to poor filling of the aorta there is poor filling of the coronary arteries, leading to myocardial ischaemia, and the left ventricle hypertrophies to overcome the valvular obstruction. These effects may combine to produce cardiac failure.

CONGENITAL HEART DISEASE

1. Cyanotic
Caused by shunting of venous (i.e. de-oxygenated) blood into the arterial circulation through an abnormal communication between the heart chambers. Usually due to failure of development of the

inter-atrial or inter-ventricular septum. Finger clubbing is often seen.

2. Acyanotic
Here there is either no abnormal mixing of arterial and venous blood or the shunt of blood flow is from the arterial side e.g. patent ductus arteriosus.

Classification:
1. *Cyanotic*
   - (i) Fallot's tetrad
     - Pulmonary stenosis
     - Ventricular septal defect (VSD)
     - Over-riding aorta
     - Right ventricular hypertrophy
   - (ii) Eisenmenger complex
     - VSD with pulmonary hypertension
   - (iii) Transposition of the great vessels, and tricuspid atresia are usually fatal in infancy
2. *Acyanotic*
   - (A) With L to R shunt
     - (i) VSD
     - (ii) Atrial septal defect (ASD)
     - (iii) Persistent ductus arteriosus
   - (B) With no shunt
     - (i) Coarctation of the aorta
     - (ii) Pulmonary stenosis
     - (iii) Congenital aortic stenosis
     - (iv) Bicuspid aortic valves

All congenital malformations of the heart and great vessels predispose the patient to bacterial endocarditis, and should receive antibiotic cover for dental procedures which cause bleeding.

RHEUMATIC FEVER

Children and young adults are predominantly affected. Three main features are:
   - Fever
   - Arthritis
   - Carditis

The carditis may result in permanent damage to the heart valves. Frequently starts with a sore throat due to β-haemolytic streptococci of Lancefield group A. This organism may have a common antigen with a component of connective tissue and thus the diverse effects on heart and joints result from an immunological response evoked by the streptococci. The characteristic histopathological feature is the *Aschoff node* seen throughout the connective tissue of the body — zone of necrosis surrounded by chronic inflammatory cells (plasma cells and lymphocytes). These inflammatory foci in the endocardium and heart valves cause damage and circulating platelets adhere to them giving *vegetations.* Subsequent fibrosis causes valvular distortion leading to stenosis or incompetence. Severe cardiac failure may occur in the acute phase of rheumatic fever.

Principles of treatment
1. Bed rest until the disease is quiescent
2. Penicillin to eliminate the streptococci
3. Salicylates (aspirin) act as an anti-inflammatory agent and also relieve the joint pains.

BACTERIAL ENDOCARDITIS

Acute bacterial endocarditis is due to bacteria such as staphylococci affecting normal valves in seriously ill patients. *Subacute bacterial endocarditis* (SABE) is a less severe disease due to *Streptococcus viridans,* which attacks previously damaged valves.

Oral commensals (such as *Strep. viridans*) enter the cirulation when bleeding occurs during dental procedures or even during normal mastication in mouths with chronic periodontal disease.

Impeccable oral health is very important for patients at risk from bacterial endocarditis (e.g. with valvular or congenital heart disease) and antibiotic cover is required for these patients, (see Antibiotic Cover). Without antibiotic cover there is an increased risk of organisms in the circulation adhering to roughened areas of myocardium where there has been damage by valvular disease or other cause. Inflammation then results in platelet adhesions forming crumbling vegetations and the fragments which break away are carried in the circulation as emboli.

Clinical features of SABE
These are of insidious onset, which often causes delay in diagnosis. Blood culture is required to confirm diagnosis and show the causal organisms together with its antibiotic sensitivity. Several cultures are often required. The features of SABE are:
1. Septicaemia
2. Endocarditis
3. Embolism

1. *SEPTICAEMIA* causes intermittent *pyrexia, anaemia* (manifest as pallor) or a *'cafe-au-lait'* tint to the skin in advanced cases, and *splenomegaly.*

2. *ENDOCARDITIS* with murmurs, as the valvular lesions develop or become more severe. The decreased efficiency of such a damaged heart, with anaemia and toxaemia, may lead to cardiac failure. Finger clubbing is frequently present.
3. *EMBOLISM* from the crumbling vegetations in the heart lesion. The most important sites affected are:
   a) *Skin and conjunctiva* — Petechial haemorrhages. Small (splinter) haemorrhages under the fingernails are common. *Osler's Nodes* (pink tender swellings at finger tips) are seen
   b) *Kidney* — multiple small infarcts give the kidney a 'flea-bitten' appearance. The damage also allows red blood cells to appear in urine.
   c) *Retina* — blockage of the retinal artery causes immediate blindness in the affected eye
   d) *Spleen* — infarction causes the spleen to become enlarged and tender
   e) *Brain* — cerebral embolism with loss of function of the area of cerebral cortex affected e.g. contralateral hemiplegia
   f) *Mesenteric arteries* — may become blocked producing paralysis of that portion of gut, leading to intestinal obstruction

Treatment
1. Bed rest
2. Intense, prolonged antibiotic therapy based upon blood culture sensitivity results. The duration of antibiotic therapy is often 6 or more weeks.
3. Complications of embolism or cardiac failure are treated as they arise

Prognosis
Until the advent of antibiotics this disease was invariably fatal, due to cardiac failure or embolism.

Prevention and prophylaxis
Careful history taking from patients to discover a previous history of valvular or rheumatic heart disease or congenital heart disease. Any patient with such a history must receive antibiotic cover prior to any dental procedure which causes bleeding.

ANTIBIOTIC COVER

It is important to remember the following factors in choosing antibiotic cover:
1. The antibacterial drug MUST be bactericidal (thus tetracyclines which are bacteriostatic are totally unsuitable)
2. The drug MUST be given *immediately* pre-operatively and *not* 24 or more hours pre-operatively

3. Sufficiently high blood levels of drug must be attained and maintained for sufficiently long post-operatively

Patients requiring antibiotic cover fall into one of the following four categories:

(A) Those on long-term prophylactic penicillin
(B) Those who have had penicillin within 2 months of the proposed dental procedure
(C) Those allergic to penicillin
(D) Those able to have penicillin (i.e. not allergic to it, not on long-term penicillin and not having received penicillin within 2 months for any other reason).

Suitable antibiotic cover regimes

Category D
At present *penicillin* is the drug of choice and most cases fall into category D, above. For penicillin antibiotic cover:
Age 12 years or above — 600 mg crystalline penicillin with 300 mg procaine penicillin *intramuscularly 30 minutes* pre-operatively, followed by 250 mg phenoxymethyl-penicillin orally every 6 hours for 3 days minimum post-operatively.

Intramuscular injection ensures absorption of the penicillin so that effective blood levels are present when the dental operation is performed. Where intramuscular injection is impossible (very rare indeed) 2 gm phenoxymethyl-penicillin orally *2 hours* pre-operatively is a less certain alternative to be followed by 250 mg phenoxymethyl-penicillin orally every 6 hours for a minimum of 3 days post-operatively.

It has recently been suggested that a pulse dose of 3 gm amoxycillin orally 1 hour pre-operatively gives sufficient antibiotic cover pre- and post-operatively for dental procedures in those patients of group D. For this purpose, amoxycillin is presented pre-packed in a sachet and the 3 gm contents are dissolved in a glass of water and drunk 1 hour pre-operatively.

Amoxycillin, being a penicillin, *cannot* be used for the penicillin allergic patient.

Oral loading doses are contraindicated when general anaesthesia is used and intramuscular loading is then employed where applicable.
Age under 12 years — The above dose regimes are halved.

Patients of groups A, B, and C
Age 12 years or over — 100 mg erythromycin by deep intramuscular injection in a large muscle ½-hour pre-operatively.
Less certain, where injection *is impossible*, 2 gm erythromycin tablets may be given 2 hours pre-operatively.

This is to be followed in each case by 250 mg erythromycin orally every 6 hours for 3 days minimum.
NB NOT erythromycin estolate as this drug may cause severe liver damage.
Age under 12 years — Halve the above dosages.
In rare cases (if managed properly) where a patient is both allergic to penicillin and has had erythromycin therapy within 2 months of the proposed dental treatment, an alternative is 2 gm clindamycin orally 2 hours pre-operatively followed by 250 mg clindamycin orally every 6 hours for 3 days minimum. Clindamycin is, however, closely associated with *pseudomembranous colitis* due to overgrowth of *Clostridia* in the bowel which are resistant to clindamycin. This serious complication cannot be predicted and may be fatal even after short courses of therapy with this drug. Its general use is, therefore, not advised. For children under 12 years of age the above dosages should be halved.

Patients of groups A and B
In these patients there is no hypersensitivity (allergy) to penicillin and some authorities recommend using cephaloridine compounds as antibiotic cover. For these cases 500 mg cephaloridine should be given i.m. 30 min pre-operatively followed by 250 mg Cephalexin ® Caps every 6 hours for 3 days minimum. Children under 12 years of age should receive half the above dosages.
Note:
1. Cephaloridines frequently show cross-hypersensitivity with penicillin so may not be used in the penicillin allergic patient with safety.
2. Cephaloridines may cause renal damage and should not be used in patients with renal disease.
Note:
Antibiotic cover regimes vary from region to region in this country and reflect local bacterial susceptibility to antibiotics (probably representing the prescribing habits of medical, dental and veterinary practitioners) as well as the varying opinions of local physicians and bacteriologists. Advice from these local authorities should be sought in uncertain situations. The regimes advocated here reflect the current opinions in Bristol United Hospitals.

SUMMARY OF SUB-ACUTE BACTERIAL ENDOCARDITIS

Occurs in patients with pre-existing heart disease
Caused by bacteraemia, e.g. following dental procedures which cause bleeding
Features of the disease are:
1 Low-grade fever and malaise
2. Changing heart murmurs

3. Anaemia (inc. 'Cafe-au-lait' appearance in severe cases)
4. Finger-clubbing and splinter nail-bed haemorrhages
5. Other embolic complications e.g. haematuria
6. End result may be cardiac failure and death
Treatment 6 weeks effective antibiotic therapy and bed rest.

Prophylaxis
1. History taking by dental surgeon to identify patients at risk, and consultation with physicians where indicated
2. Effective bactericidal *antibiotic cover*. Penicillin is the drug of choice, at pesent

FINGER CLUBBING

This easily recognised clinical sign should never be missed. The tissue around the base of the nails of the fingers, and often toes, becomes thickened causing the ends of the phalanges to become enlarged and club-shaped, with curved nails and filling-in of the angle at the nail base. The mechanism by which this occurs is obscure.

Common causes of clubbing

Respiratory
1. Bronchial carcinoma
2. Chronic pulmonary suppuration

Cardiovascular
1. Bacterial endocarditis
2. Cyanotic congenital heart disease

Less common causes include:
1. Asbestosis, especially with mesothelioma
2. Fibrosing alveolitis
3. Ulcerative colitis
4. Crohn's disease

PULMONARY HEART DISEASE

Cor pulmonale
Cardiac disease secondary to disease of lungs or pulmonary vessels.
1. Chronic pulmonary fibrosis may occlude the pulmonary vasculature, and the associated pulmonary hypertension gives rise to right-sided heart failure
2. Chronic bronchitis and emphysema

3. Pulmonary emboli: sudden obstruction of pulmonary circulation by embolis, may follow from migration of thrombus in leg through circulation via R side of heart. Deep vein thrombosis of the legs may follow immobilisation in bed following general surgery or childbirth with the resultant risk of acute cor pulmonale.

ARTERIAL DISEASE

1. Atheroma
Patchy degenerative process resulting in thickened plaques in the intima of arteries. Closely associated with hypertension and increasing age. Secondary damage to the arterial media frequently follows. Lumen of vessel becomes narrowed leading to arterial insufficiency of the region supplied, and thrombosis arising on the roughened intimal surface of the vessel.

Atheroma formation may be increased by genetic predisposition, cigarette smoking, diabetes, hypertension and ingestion of animal fat (saturated fats) in excess.

The main vessels affected with serious consequences are:
a. *Coronary arteries* — angina of effort, myocardial infarction or sudden death.
b. *Cerebral arteries* — blackouts, dementia, thrombosis or haemorrhage (stroke).
c. *Iliac or lower limb vessels* — cramping pains in the feet and calves, due to muscle ischaemia. Pain is relieved by rest (cf. angina) and made worse by using the affected muscles, e.g. by walking (intermittent claudication).
d. *Renal vessels* — leads to renal ischaemia which itself activates the renin/angiotensin system leading to increased blood pressure. The hypertension will promote further atheroma, thus producing a vicious circle.

2. Senile arterial disease
Senile hardening of arterial vessel walls. There may be intramural calcification of the arteries visible on radiographs (Mönckeberg's sclerosis) but these changes by themselves do no alter the patency of the arterial lumen and are of little clinical importance. Atheroma may also be present and will cause symptoms of ischaemia.

3. Syphilitic aortic disease

Has a predilection for the thoracic aorta and leads to destruction of the muscular and elastic tissue in the arterial wall (tunica media). The lesion is repaired by fibrous tissue, which results in one or more of the following:

a. Aortic aneurysm
b. Aortic incompetence
c. Occlusion of opening of coronary vessels

4. Aortic aneurysm

Due to syphilis when the thoracic aorta is involved, or atheroma when the abdominal aorta is affected. The effects of the aneurysm result from the enlarged pulsating mass which results, e.g.

a. Dysphagia due to pressure on the oesophagus
b. Cough and dyspnoea due to pressure on the trachea
c. Pain due to erosion of vertebrae
d. Pulsatile swelling in either the abdomen or chest wall

A *dissecting* aneurysm is an uncommon condition in which the tunica media of the aorta degenerates and blood escapes from the vessel lumen into the space between the tunica intima and tunica externa of the aorta. This causes collapse and sudden severe chest pain similar to that due to myocardial infarction. Death usually ensues in a few hours.

Rupture of an aortic aneurysm usually results in sudden death.

5. Vasomotor arterial disease

Raynaud's phenomenon is a condition in which increased sensitivity to cold results in severe spasm of the arteries of the fingers. Women are most frequently affected. When the vasospasm occurs the fingers become white, then cyanotic and later turn red as a result of reactive hyperaemia. There may be associated numbness, tingling, or pain. In severe cases gangrene may occur. The condition may be associated with serious systemic disease such as systemic sclerosis, or it may occur as an isolated finding. Treatment involves protection against cold, systemic vasodilators or in severe cases cervical sympathectomy.

DISEASES OF VEINS

Thrombosis and thrombophlebitis

A thrombus is a solid blood clot formed within a vessel. Factors which predispose to thrombosis are:

a. Increased coaguability of blood — e.g. following major surgery, injuries which involve blood loss, or childbirth
b. Stasis of blood — frequently associated with immobilisation. Major surgery thus produces a severe risk of deep vein thrombosis, especially in the legs. Early post-surgical mobilisation is an important preventive measure.

c. Damage to vessel walls. This may result from external trauma, or injury inside the vessels e.g. from intravenous needles or catheters, for infusion of fluid or drugs. The combination of trauma and irritant drugs in this situation may cause inflammation of the vein (phlebitis) which predisposes to venous thrombosis (thrombophlebitis).

Venous thrombosis

Clinical features
Tenderness and distal swelling. In superficial thrombophlebitis the overlying skin is red.
Complications
Pulmonary embolism, due to detachment of a clot which enters the pulmonary circulation.

Cavernous sinus thrombosis
May arise from infection in the middle third of the face, the infective material being carried via the inferior ophthalmic veins (no valves) to the intra-cranial cavernous sinus. Such infections may result from dental disease or maxillary skeletal fractures. Effective antibiotic therapy is required for this dangerous condition which may be fatal despite these measures. Cavernous sinus thrombosis with subsequent meningitis and death has arisen from a small particle of calculus landing in a dental surgeon's eye during normal scaling and polishing. The importance of eye protection in Dentistry cannot be over-emphasized.

Arterial thrombosis
Clinic features depend on the site affected, but there is generally *ischaemia* which produces loss of function or necrosis of the affected area. Blockage of a main artery to a limb for example causes pain and the skin distal to the block becomes pale and cold, and may eventually develop gangrene.

DENTAL PRACTICE AND CARDIOVASCULAR DISEASE

Summary
Cardiac disease is very common and every dental surgeon MUST be aware of his responsibility towards the correct management of these patients in dental practice.

1. Cardiac failure
Serious risk from general anaesthesia — not to be undertaken by a dentist. Local analgesia is preferred. By far the most important and common symptom is **breathlessness.**

2. Cyanosis

A definite contraindication to general anaesthesia. Any patient showing cyanosis must be regarded as medically unfit and any form of dental treatment however simple should be performed with the advice of the patient's medical adviser.

3. SABE

More likely in those with a history of rheumatic fever, or other valvular or congenital heart disease, following dental procedures which produce bleeding. Adequate medical history taking is essential and the correct provision of antibiotic cover for such patients reduces the risk from dentally-induced bacteraemia.

4. Hypertension

Again, general anaesthesia in the dental chair is absolutely contraindicated. Local analgesia is safe though some would recommend the use of adrenaline-free local analgesic preparations. A suitable alternative is 3% prilocaine with felypressin (Citanest and Octapressin, Astra Pharmaceuticals, Ltd.) and in all cases the use of an aspirating syringe is essential.

5. Cerebral or coronary thrombosis

In the susceptible patient this may arise during dental procedures in the dental surgery, where pain and fear may be the precipitating factors. Urgent medical attention is required for these eventualities. Most are best avoided by correct patient assessment pre-operatively and liaison with the patient's medical adviser.

Respiratory system

LUNG VOLUMES

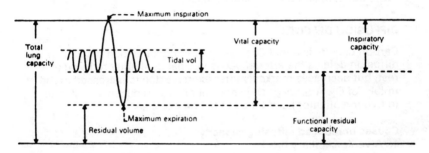

Fig. 2 Lung volumes.
(Reproduced from Burton J L 1980 Aids to undergraduate medicine, 3rd edn, with permission.)

The resting expiratory level is the most constant reference point on the spirometer tracing.

Minute ventilation — product of tidal volume and number of respirations per minute.

Vital capacity — largest volume a subject can expire after a single maximal inspiration. Normal values increase with size of subject and decrease with age (about 4½ litres in young adult male). Can be reduced in practically any lung or chest wall disease.

Forced vital capacity (FVC) — the vital capacity when the expiration is performed as rapidly as possible.

FEV$_1$ (Forced expiratory volume in one second) — volume expired during first second of FVC.

Ratio $\frac{FEV_1}{FVC}$ should be 75% or more, and is reduced in obstructive airway diseases (asthma, emphysema, bronchitis).

19

Peak flow — maximum expiratory flow rate achieved during a forced expiration. A convenient way to detect a reduction in ventilatory function. Also useful for serial measurements in the same patient and for assessing response to bronchial antispasmodics.

Residual volume — obtained by subtracting expiratory reserve volume from functional residual capacity. Residual volume is normally 20–25% of total lung capacity but increases in elderly, and in over-inflation of the lungs (emphysema, asthma).

Anatomical dead space — The volume of air in the mouth, pharynx, trachea and bronchi up to the terminal bronchioles (about 150 ml). In disease the physiological dead space may greatly exceed the anatomical dead space due to disorders of the ventilation/perfusion ratio, but in health the two are identical.

DIFFUSION DEFECTS

Carbon dioxide is about 20 times more diffusible than oxygen. In diffusion defects the *arterial pO_2* is normal or slightly reduced at rest, but decreases markedly after exercise due to increased tissue uptake of O_2. *Arterial pCO_2* is normal or even reduced at rest (due to hyperventilation) and tends to fall on exercise.

Causes of reduced diffusing capacity
1. Alveolo-capillary block
    (i) pulmonary oedema
    (ii) pulmonary fibrosis
    (iii) infiltrative lesions, e.g. sarcoidosis
2. Reduction in area available for diffusion
    (i) emphysema
    (ii) multiple pulmonary emboli

Lung compliance
A measure of lung elasticity. Compliance is reduced when the lungs are abnormally stiff due to pulmonary venous congestion or infiltrative or fibrotic lesions of the lungs.

BLOOD-GAS ANALYSIS

These values must be related to the normal levels expected for the subject, e.g. baby, old man, pregnant woman.

Hypoxia is oxygen deficiency at a specified site
Hypoxaemia is oxygen deficiency in the blood. In arterial blood of normal resting adult,
    pCO_2 is about 40 mmHg
    pO_2 is about 80–100 mmHg

Causes of hypoxaemia
1. Cardio-respiratory discorders
    (i) Hypoventilation
    (ii) Abnormality of ventilation/perfusion ratio
    (iii) Impaired diffusion
    (iv) Venous to arterial shunt
2. Decreased pO_2 of inspired gas, e.g. high altitude
3. Reduction in active haemoglobin, e.g. coal gas poisoning

Dyspnoea is a subjective awareness of the need for an increased respiratory effort.
Hypoventilation is a reduction in lung ventilation sufficient to cause hypercapnia.
Kussmaul's breathing (air hunger). Occurs in acidosis (uraemia, diabetes mellitus) due to stimulation of respiratory centre.
Cheyne–Stokes breathing — amplitude of respiration progressively deepens to a maximum, then decreases to a period of apnoea. Due to diminished sensitivity of respiratory centre to CO_2. Occurs in left ventricular failure, central respiratory depression and in normal infants.

DEFINITIONS OF COMMON PULMONARY DISEASES

Simple chronic bronchitis
Chronic or recurrent increase in the volume of mucoid bronchial secretion sufficient to cause expectoration.

Chronic obstructive bronchitis
Chronic bronchitis in which there is persistent widespread narrowing of the intra-pulmonary airways, at least on expiration, causing increased resistance to air flow.

Asthma
Is characterized by variable, often paroxysmal, dyspnoea due to widespread narrowing of the bronchioles.

Emphysema
Is characterized by enlargement of the air spaces distal to the terminal bronchioles, with destruction of the alveolar walls.

THE COMMON COLD (acute coryza)
Acute viral infection caused by any one of 30 different rhinoviruses as well as many types of adenoviruses. Immunity, therefore, is difficult to achieve due to the large variety of organisms.

Furthermore, viruses change their antigenic status during transmission to another host. Characterized by:
Swelling of mucosa of nose and nasopharynx
Fever
Headache
Sneezing
Nasal discharge and blockage
Cough
Malaise
Suffused eyes
Secondary bacterial infection occurs after a few days, changing the early watery secretion to a muco-purulent discharge.
Common complications include laryingitis, tracheobronchitis and otitis media.

Treatment
Bed rest, hot drinks and antipyretic analgesics (e.g. aspirin) are comforting.
Antihistamines with pseudephedrine (e.g. Actifed®) to dry-up the nasal secretions are sometimes useful. Megavitamin C therapy has not been conclusively proven to be useful.
Antibiotics for secondary bacterial infection control.

ACUTE SINUSITIS

Often follows a coryza. Due to infection of the mucosal lining of the paranasal sinuses. A thick muco-purulent discharge collects in these air spaces which have naturally poor drainage anyway. There is pain over the affected sinus and mild fever. With maxillary sinusitis, the maxillary molar teeth may be periodontitic.

Treatment
Antibiotics to control secondary infection. Antipyretic analgesics, medicated inhalations and ephedrine nose drops to shrink the swollen mucous membranes and promote drainage from the sinuses. Surgical drainage may be required.

CHRONIC SINUSITIS

Usually preceded by acute sinusitis.
There is a persistent mucopurulent discharge into the nose or nasopharynx (post-nasal drip) and headache is common.
Recurrences of acute sinusitis are common.

Treatment
Antibiotics, ephedrine nose drops and, perhaps, surgical intervention to improve the natural drainage from the sinuses.

HAY FEVER (Allergic Rhinitis)

Allergic inflammatory response in the nasal mucosa. Common antigens are pollens from grass, flowers and trees. Thus, there is a higher incidence during spring and early summer. There is episodic sneezing, watery nasal secretions and lacrimation. Does not progress to the thick muco-purulent discharge stage as seen in the common cold.

Treatment

Antihistamines orally or sodium cromoglycate insufflation. Desensitization programmes using intra-dermal injections of pollen extract are beneficial in selected cases.

TONSILLITIS

Infection of the tonsils (epithelially covered collections of lymphoid tissue in the throat).

There is variable fever, sore throat with pain on swallowing, and headache and vomiting may occur, especially in children. Tonsils are enlarged, with a creamy exudate and enlarged anterior cervical lymph glands.

Often viral in origin. An important bacterial cause is infection with β-haemolytic streptococci of Lancefield's Group A, which may also cause scarlet fever, acute glomerulonephritis or rheumatic fever. Diagnosis is by culture and antibiotic sensitivity testing of the bacteria obtained from a throat swab.

Treatment

For β-haemolytic streptococcal infections, intramuscular penicillin is used to ensure effective eradication of the organism and prevent complications such as nephritis or rheumatic fever. Bed rest, gargles and antipyretic analgesics are comforting.

SORE THROAT

This is a common symptom of upper respiratory tract infections. Important specific conditions are:

1. Streptococcal or viral tonsillitis

2. Glandular fever (Infective Mononucleosis)
This viral disease is characterized by mild fever, malaise, sore throat and marked regional lymphadenopathy. There are characteristic abnormal white cells seen on blood films.
The acute phase lasts for 2–3 weeks but there may be a prolonged period of convalescence. Hepatomegaly with jaundice may occur as well as splenomegaly and a rash.
This disease can lead to false positive W.R. serology.

3. Blood dyscrasias
Here malfunction or absence of white cells leads to spreading widespread infection. The throat is an early target. This is seen in acute leukaemia, aplastic anaemia and agranulocytosis.

4. Vincent's angina
A rare form of ulcerative pharyngitis due to *Borellia vincenti* and *Bacillus fusiformis*, identifiable in stained smears of throat swabs. Oral metronidazole therapy is an effective antimicrobial therapy. Obstruction of the airway requires urgent hospital attention.

5. Diphtheria
Throat and tonsils infected with *Corynebacterium diphtheriae*, identifiable in stained smears of throat swabs. A grey adherent slough covers the tonsils (diphtheric membrane). When this involves the larynx death from choking can occur. This serious disease is now rare in UK due to immunization.

LARYNGITIS

Acute laryngitis often accompanies upper respiratory tract infections, including coryza. Dry painful cough with hoarseness and loss of voice.

Chronic laryngitis
Common in actors, teachers or others who use their voice for prolonged periods. Chronic infectious disease of the larynx is uncommon (e.g. tuberculosis or syphilis). Important causes of chronic hoarseness are carcinoma of the larynx or paralysis of the vocal cords.
Chronic hoarseness requires laryngoscopy to establish the diagnosis.

Treatment
Resting the voice and analgesic therapy is often all that is required. For bacterial infections a suitable antibiotic should be administered.

LARYNGEAL OBSTRUCTION

More common in children, in whom the larynx is smaller.
1. Inhalation of foreign body e.g. tooth, sweet
2. Laryngeal spasm — due to irritation e.g. noxious fumes. Some drugs tend to produce laryngeal spasm, e.g. ether and intravenous barbiturates
3. Oedema — either inflammatory or allergic (angio-oedema)
4. Diphtheria — almost unknown in UK today

Treatment
Removal of foreign body. Emergency treatment may require establishing an airway below the level of obstruction (tracheostomy). For laryngeal spasm administer oxygen and if possible remove cause. In inflammatory conditions, control oedema with steroids and antibiotic therapy where indicated.

DISEASES OF THE BRONCHIAL TREE

Cough
Common symptom of bronchial and tracheal disease. Nature and quality of the sputum produced is useful in making a diagnosis.
Dry cough — may be nervous in origin or due to excessive smoking. Also a feature of early pneumonia or tuberculosis, acute bronchitis or viral infections, e.g. influenza or common cold.
Productive cough — may indicate infection, where there is a variable mixture of mucus and pus. This is characteristic of chronic bronchitis and the later stages of acute bronchitis. Bronchiectasis often produces foul-smelling muco-purulent sputum.
In all these inflammatory conditions blood vessels may become damaged and red blood streaks will appear in the sputum (haemoptysis). In tuberculosis there is scanty sputum and cough at first. Later, large amounts of muco-purulent blood-stained sputum are produced and the cough is pronounced and exhausting.
Left-sided heart disease (e.g. mitral stenosis and cardiac failure) often causes coughing. Pulmonary oedema due to left ventricular failure is associated with large volumes of pink frothy sputum, the pinkness being due to blood.

Acute bronchitis
Common disease affecting all ages. Often follows influenza, common cold, measles or whooping-cough. Cough is at first dry, irritating and non-productive. Fever, headache and malaise with aching limbs are characteristic, especially where there is a viral cause. Later, cough becomes productive with yellow muco-purulent sputum. Bronchial obstruction occurs giving a wheeziness to the breath sounds. Dry sounds (rhonchi) or moist sounds (rales) may be heard over the lung fields with a stethoscope. In the elderly or debilitated, broncho-pneumonia may develop. This may cause pulmonary hypertension and lead to right ventricular failure.

Treatment
Consists of bed rest, aspirin, a cough mixture with codeine to control coughing spasms and antibiotics such as trimethoprim-sulphamethoxazole to control secondary bacterial infection.

Chronic bronchitis

Commonest respiratory disease in Britain, due to smoking, atmospheric pollution and the cool damp climate. Middle-aged and elderly are more commonly affected.
There is cough, and increasing disability due to dyspnoea (breathlessness). Acute exacerbations are frequent. The sputum may be mucoid in the chronic stage but pus-stained in the acute phases. Wheezing is prominent due to obstruction of bronchi and bronchospasm (asthma). Dry sounds (rhonchi) and moist sounds (rales) are heard with the stethoscope. Broncho-pneumonia and pulmonary heart disease are common complications.

Treatment
Expectorant mixtures to try and remove viscid secretions, with oral or inhaled bronchodilators (e.g. aminophylline) to relax bronchospasm. Purulent sputum is an indication for antibiotics (e.g. ampicillin or amoxycillin).
Physiotherapy with postural drainage is helpful.
Chronic oral disease and sepsis should be eliminated.

Asthma

Asthma is characterized by attacks of severe breathlessness (dyspnoea) accompanied by wheezing. Bronchospasm makes exhalation difficult but inhalation is relatively unaffected. Thus, the lungs are full of air, making the chest barrel-shaped. The strenuous efforts made by the patient to empty the lungs may be exhausting. The attacks are often of sudden onset and may last for an hour or much longer. Between attacks the patient may be well, but in long-established cases infection and emphysema develop.
The condition often starts in childhood. The following may be relevant influencing factors:
1. Infection of the bronchial tree
2. Allergy to dusts, pollen, animal hair may be precipitating factors in sensitive subjects. Desensitization injections may be useful.
3. Psychological factors such as anxiety or stress.

Severe prolonged attacks (status asthmaticus) may cause the patient to become cyanosed. There may be loss of consciousness and even death. Such acute attacks are treated with intravenous steroids or bronchodilators, such as aminophylline.

EMPHYSEMA

Here the lungs have lost their elasticity due to recurrent infection and fibrotic repair of the damaged pulmonary epithelium. The alveolar walls break down and form distended air spaces.
Frequently associated with chronic bronchitis and asthma.
Due to the fibrosis and loss of alveolar epithelium, oxygen transfer

across the lungs to the pulmonary blood is hindered. Thus, there is increasing incapacity of the patient with breathlessness. Broncho-pneumonia often occurs in such damaged lungs.

Treatment
Physiotherapy to improve pulmonary ventilation and remove any mucoid material. Acute respiratory infections require antibiotic therapy. Emphysema is often progressive and defies treatment.

Causes of emphysema

Localized
1. Congenital
2. Compensatory, due to lung collapse, scarring or resection
3. Partial bronchial occlusion
    (i) foreign body
    (ii) neoplasm
    (iii) peribronchial lymphadenopathy

Generalized
1. Idiopathic ('primary')
2. Secondary to chronic bronchitis
                        chronic asthma
                        or pneumoconiosis
3. Senile (physiological)
4. Rarely familial (some due to an anti-trypsin deficiency)

BLOCKAGE OF A BRONCHUS

This may arise in one of three ways (like all obstructions to a hollow organ):

1. Blockage of the lumen
This may be by inhalation of a foreign body e.g. tooth, sweet or blood. Food or vomit may be inhaled by an unconscious patient. Foreign bodies such as teeth usually come to rest in the *right* bronchus as this is more vertical than the left bronchus.

2. Swelling in the wall of the bronchus
The commonest cause is carcinoma of the bronchus.

3. Space-occupying lesion outside the bronchus
e.g. enlarged lymph nodes or aortic aneurysm.

The complications of bronchus blockage are:

1. *Collapse of part of lung*
Air beyond the obstruction is absorbed into the blood stream, and the affected part is then not refilled during breathing. If the part affected is large there is dyspnoea, and cyanosis. If small, there may be no symptoms.

2. *Infection* may develop in the non-ventilated portion of lung.

3. *Abscess formation* may occur subsequent to the infection as drainage is not possible.

4. *Bronchiectasis* results from the mixture of obstruction and infection which causes the weakened smaller bronchi to dilate and form sac-like bulges.

Treatment
Surgical removal of the obstruction. Antibiotic therapy is indicated, and an abscess may need surgical drainage.

BRONCHIECTASIS

Dilation of the bronchi, usually accompanied by recurrent bronchial suppuration.

Pathogenesis
Increased outward traction on the bronchi and weakness of the bronchial wall due to inflammation are both important.

Causes
1. Infection
   (i) Bronchiolitis of infancy
   (ii) Measles or pertussis in children
   (iii) Post broncho-pneumonic collapse in adults
   (iv) Commonly in post-primary TB, but apical; therefore secondary infection is unusual
2. Bronchial stenosis or occlusion
   (i) Adenoma or carcinoma
   (ii) Foreign body or asthma casts
   (iii) Lymphadenopathy
3. Pulmonary aspergillosis
4. Mucoviscidosis
5. Congenital
6. Many cases are idiopathic

Clinical features
1. Classical symptom — cough with copious purulent sputum, especially on changing posture
2. Classical sign — localized persistent coarse crepitations
3. May be asymptomatic
4. Malaise, intermittent fever, halitosis
5. Weight loss or 'failure to thrive'
6. Dyspnoea, cyanosis or clubbing
7. Haemoptysis ('dry bronchiectasis')
8. Signs of collapse or fibrosis
9. Coexisting chronic sinusitis is common

Complications
1. Recurrent pneumonia after upper respiratory infection
2. Recurrent dry pleurisy
3. Massive haemoptysis
4. Lung abscess, empyema or cerebral abscess
5. Cor pulmonale
6. Amyloidosis

PNEUMONIA

Anatomical classification

1. Lobar
Due to virulent organisms such as 'epidemic' pneumococcus (e.g. Type 3).,
Staphylococcus aureus or Friedlander's (*Klebsiella*)

2. Segmental ('Benign aspiration pneumonia')
Due to organisms of low virulence
Often follows upper respiratory tract infections

3. Lobular ('Bronchopneumonia' if bilateral)
Occurs in babies and elderly or debilitated patients. Due to *Haemophilus influenzae*, 'carrier' pneumococci, streptococci, TB.

Aetiological classification

1. Infective
  (i) Bacterial (see above)
Pneumonia may also be a feature of generalized bacterial infections, e.g. brucellosis, typhoid fever, plague.
  (ii) Viral
     Ornithosis
     Respiratory syncytial
     Influenza (usually with secondary bacterial infection)

Mumps (usually secondary bacterial infection)
Cytomegalovirus
URT viruses (adenovirus, rhinovirus, parainfluenza)
(iii) Rickettsial
Typhus
Q fever
(iv) Mycoplasmal
M-pneumoniae (Eaton agent)
(v) Yeasts and fungi
Candida
Actinomyces
Histoplasma
(vi) Protozoa and parasites
Toxoplasma
Amoebae
Pneumocystis carinii
2. Allergic
Collagen-vascular disease (esp. polyarteritis nodosa)
Stevens-Johnson syndrome (Erythema multiforme)
3. Chemical agents
(i) Irritant gases: NH_3, SO_2, Cl, oxides of nitrogen
(ii) Irritant liquids
Vomitus
Lipoid pneumonia
4. Physical agents
Irradiation

In discussing causes of pneumonia remember the possibility of
1. Pre-existing lung disease, e.g. bronchial carcinoma,
bronchiectasis
2. Inhalation pneumonia
(i) Oral and pharyngeal sepsis and sinusitis
(ii) Oesophageal obstruction and pharyngeal pouch
(iii) Alcoholic debauch, drowning or anaesthesia
(iv) Laryngeal cancer
(v) Tracheo-oesophageal fistula
3. Predisposing systemic disease such as diabetes, cirrhosis or
agranulocytosis
4. Foreign body not seen on X-ray (e.g. peanut)

Complications of pneumococcal lobar pneumonia
1. Pleurisy with effusion, or serous pericarditis
2. Empyema or pericardial suppuration
3. Endocarditis, septicaemia, meningitis (not to be confused with
meningismus, in which c.s.f. is normal) or cerebral abscess.
4. Delayed resolution

5. Nonspecific complications
    (i) Herpes labialis
    (ii) Paralytic ileus
    (iii) Jaundice
    (iv) Shock
    (v) Cardiac failure, sometimes with arrhythmia
    (vi) Deep vein thrombosis

Signs of diffuse airways obstruction and lung distension
1. Inspection
    (i) Increased AP diameter of chest
    (ii) Excavation of supra-clavicular fossae during inspiration
    (iii) Jugular venous filling during expiration
2. Palpation
    (i) Use of accessory muscles
    (ii) Tracheal descent with inspiration
    (iii) Paradoxical movement of costal margin
3. Percussion
    Decreased heart and liver dullness
4. Auscultation
    (i) Diminished breath sounds
    (ii) Forced expiratory time exceeds 4 seconds

TUBERCULOSIS

Bacteriology
Caused by the rod-shaped organism *Mycobacterium tuberculosis*.
Demonstrated by the Ziehl-Neelsen staining technique in smears.
The bacterium can survive for long periods in dry conditions due to
its waxy envelope. The pathological process is the result of an
allergic-type response to a protein in this waxy envelope.

Pathology
Initial contact with the bacillus produces an inflammatory
reaction — the *tubercular follicle*. This consists of a collection of
reticulo-endothelial cells which become infiltrated with giant cells
and surrounded by lymphocytes. Necrosis (caseation) occurs in the
centre of this follicle. Coalescence of follicles like this causes a
small, visible lump to form, giving the characteristic *tubercle* from
which the disease derives its name.

PRIMARY TUBERCULOSIS

This is the reaction seen in a person who has never before been in
contact with the bacillus.
In the lung, the primary lesion forms just beneath the pleura.
Lymphatic spread leads to the hilar lymph nodes becoming
affected which undergo caseation. The original lesion remains

inconspicuous. Gut primary lesions are the same with the regional abdominal lymph notes undergoing caseation.

The initial focus and subsequent regional lymph node involvement together form the PRIMARY COMPLEX.

Clinical features

Often very little, though there may be a 'flu-like' episode or weight loss. Also, primary TB does *not* show up on abdominal X-ray unless calcified later on. Pleural effusion may occur, and in children there is often marked enlargement of the mediastinal lymph nodes which then cause bronchial obstruction.

Fate of the Primary Lesion

1. *Healing* by fibrosis and calcification. In the lung this Ghon Focus (i.e. a calcific scar in a lung field, just beneath the pleurae) may be seen on a radiograph. This is the most common result.
2. *Tuberculous broncho-pneumonia* occurs when a follicle ruptures into a bronchus, infecting other parts of the lung. There is fever, sweating and cough. Before effective antituberculous drug therapy this was usually fatal. The infected sputum spreads the disease.
3. *Miliary tuberculosis* due to a follicle discharging its contents into a blood vessel. The bacillus is therefore spread throughout the entire body. The multiple small tubercles resemble millet seeds — thus the name. When spread in this manner to the brain tuberculous meningitis occurs. Until effective chemotherapy miliary TB was invariably fatal.
4. *Solitary or 'surgical' tuberculosis* again due to blood spread of the bacillus but where only a few organisms involved. Solitary distant lesions occurred and surgery used to be the only treatment e.g. bone tuberculosis or kidney tuberculosis.

POST — PRIMARY TUBERCULOSIS

Having once been infected, subsequent contact with the tuberculous bacillus produces a different reaction, due to both allergy and immunity.

Allergy to the protein in the envelope of the bacillus develops about six weeks after primary infection. The circulating antibodies may be demonstrated by the skin reaction to an extract of the tubercule bacillus ('tuberculin'). A raised red papule develops at the site of intracutaneous inoculation in this test. This is the *Mantoux* test.

Immunity follows primary infection with tuberculosis but this is often *incomplete*. However, this remains an important factor in the control of the disease by BCG vaccination. Today, all people who are Mantoux-negative should receive such vaccination. A specially prepared low-virulence tubercle bacillus (Bacille Calmette-Guérin) is used to give a controlled primary response.

Re-infection with tubercle bacillus or breakdown of an original healed primary lesion (such as can occur following prolonged steroid therapy) produces a different type of lesion. In the lung the lesion is usually at the lung apex. There is no regional lymph node involvement. Considerable destruction of the affected lung occurs with caseation. Bacilli enter the bronchi and are coughed up in the sputum ('open tuberculosis'). Spread of the disease readily occurs to others. Fibrotic repair tissue is laid down. There is continued destruction. When the rate of destruction does not outstrip the rate of repair, a chronic slowly progressive disease occurs — chronic fibroid phthisis. Where destruction outstrips fibrotic repair, a rapidly spreading disease results.

Clinical features
Increased pulse rate, weight loss and pyrexia (often with nocturnal sweating). Later cough and dyspnoea occur. Chest X-rays show lung apex shadows due to the cavitation. If the cavitation involves blood vessels, haemoptysis will occur.

Fate of the post-primary lesion
1. May heal
2. May spread locally with caseation and cavitation
3. Rarely, may erode a blood vessel and cause miliary tuberculosis.

Treatment
Effective chemotherapy is available but problems still arise if patients fail to take the tablets. Suitable drugs are PAS (Para-amino-salicylic acid), isoniazid (isonicotinic acid hydrazide), rifampicin, ethambutol and ethionamide. Streptomycin is now rarely used because of the risk of VIII nerve damage. More than one drug is usually used to reduce the risk of bacterial resistance developing. Treatment continues for one, two or more years. Surgical treatment e.g. lobectomy, *is now much less common due to chemotherapy.*

Causes of pulmonary collapse
1. *Absorption collapse* (due to complete bronchial obstruction)
   (i) Intraluminal, e.g. foreign body, mucus or clot
   (ii) Mural, e.g. bronchial carcinoma or adenoma
   (iii) Extramural, e.g. peribronchial lymphadenopathy or aortic aneurysm
2. *Pneumothorax or pleural effusion*

Remember that in absorption collapse the mediastinum shifts to the affected side, but in collapse due to air or fluid in the pleural space the mediastinum may shift to the opposite side.

Causes of pleural effusion

(A) Transudate (less than 2 g protein/100 ml fluid)
1. Cardiac failure
2. Nephrotic syndrome
3. Hepatic failure

(B) Exudate (more than 2 g protein/100 ml fluid)
1. Pneumonia
2. Malignancy (Bronchial Ca, secondary Ca or Hodgkin's)
3. TB
4. Pulmonary infarction
5. Collagen-vascular disease (especially SLE)
6. Subphrenic abscess

Causes of pneumothorax
1. Traumatic
2. Iatrogenic, e.g. thoracentesis or surgery
3. Spontaneous
   (i) Subpleural bulla
   (ii) Emphysema
   (iii) Asthma
   (iv) TB
   (v) Lung abscess
   (vi) Pneumoconiosis

Causes of empyema
1. Pneumonia, especially lobar, or secondary to bronchial Ca
2. Lung abscess
3. Subphrenic abscess
4. Mediastinal sepsis
5. Chest wound or surgery
6. TB

Causes of acute pulmonary oedema
1. Left heart failure
   Atrial, e.g. mitral stenosis
   Ventricular, e.g. hypertension or myocardial infarct
2. Overload of IV fluid
3. Inhalation of irritant gas, e.g. chlorine
4. Fulminating viral or bacterial pneumonia
5. Fat emboli

Common causes of haemoptysis
Exclude spurious haemoptysis (nasal bleeding, etc)

Respiratory
1. Bronchial carcinoma
2. Pulmonary tuberculosis
3. Bronchitis
4. Bronchiectasis
5. Lung abscess

Cardiovascular
1. Pulmonary infarct
2. Mitral stenosis
3. Acute left ventricular failure

Less common causes include:
1. Pneumonia, especially pneumococcal
2. Collagen-vascular disease, especially polyarteritis nodosa
3. Idiopathic pulmonary haemosiderosis

In many patients with a small haemoptysis and negative physical findings no cause is ever found despite follow-up with serial chest X-rays.

PULMONARY FIBROSIS

Caused by long-standing chronic infection or by inhalation of certain dusts.

Chronic infection produces fibrosis which, if extensive enough, can replace large amounts of normal lung tissue. Frequently associated with bronchiectasis. The distortion following fibrosis causes the lung, mediastinum and even the chest wall to become distorted. Inhalation of dusts can cause chronic inflammation and fibrosis. The most important of these dusts is silica, producing silicosis. It is guarded against today by the legal requirement to protect employees by masks etc. Stonemasons and users of grinding wheels were common sufferers, also coal miners, especially those involved with anthracite. Asbestos workers have the additional risk of a type of carcinoma (mesothelioma).

Clinical features
Increasing breathlessness and cyanosis. Increased tendency to respiratory infection is common.

Treatment
Treatment of the established condition is difficult, and prevention is important. Antibiotics to control secondary infection, where indicated.

BENIGN PULMONARY TUMOURS

Rare. Adenoma of the bronchus is the commonest type. It may be removed surgically.

MALIGNANT PULMONARY TUMOURS

1. Primary

Bronchial carcinoma
One of the commonest forms of cancer. Occurs more frequently in males, though the incidence in women is increasing. Maximum incidence in the 50–60 year old age group. Much more common in cigarette smokers.
Malignant change in the bronchial epithelium cells gives rise to a poorly differentiated tumour. The bronchus usually becomes blocked and there is collapse of that portion of lung beyond the obstruction.
Clinical features. Persistent cough and increasing dyspnoea. When collapse of a portion of lung occurs there may be resulting infection and pain of pleural origin (stabbing) with pneumonia of the collapsed lung. This never fully resolves. Haemoptysis is a very important symptom due to bleeding from the ulcerating surface of the tumour. Secondary metastases may be the first sign of bronchial carcinoma and they occur in bones, (including the mandible) and in the liver, lymph nodes, brain and elsewhere.
Treatment is by surgery, chemotherapy and radiotherapy, but the prognosis is poor in most cases.

2. Secondary malignant lung tumours

There may arise from epithelial tissue (carcinomata) or connective tissue (sarcomata). They are not uncommon in the lung and the primary sites are usually breast, kidney, thyroid gland or a primary tumour in the lung itself. Sarcomata, especially of bone, commonly metastasize to the lung. Metastases often form 'cannonball' deposits seen on chest X-ray.

Treatment
Palliative surgery, chemotherapy and radiotherapy is all that is possible.

SUPERIOR VENA CAVAL SYNDROME

A large tumour in the mediastinum may compress the superior vena cava. The resulting venous congestion is seen as neck vein distension, cyanosis and oedema of the upper half od the body.

The superficial veins in the chest wall become distended and visible as they form a collateral circulation to by-pass the caval obstruction.
Other space-occupying masses in the chest may also be a cause of superior vena caval obstruction, e.g. enlarged lymph nodes in Hodgkin's disease.

Oxygen therapy
In chronic hypoxia due to hypoventilation (e.g. chronic bronchitis, asthma), the arterial pCO_2 is raised and correction of the hypoxia by oxygen in high concentration may release the respiratory centre from its 'anoxic drive' and produce CO_2 narcosis.
Low-concentration oxygen masks such as the Venti-mask or Edinburgh mask should be used, with serial blood gas analyses.
In hypoxia due to impaired gas exchange (e.g. pneumonia, pulmonary oedema), high concentration masks such as the Polymask are required.

DENTAL ASPECTS OF RESPIRATORY DISEASE

1. *Maxillary sinusitis* may give periodontitic maxillary molar teeth
2. *Laryngeal obstruction* may result from inhalation of a foreign body during G.A. and should be prevented by correct throat packing.
3. *Blockage of a bronchus* can result from inhalation of objects during dental procedures. Where possible these may be prevented by correct use of instruments or in G.A. cases by correct throat packing, e.g. use of rubber dam when using root canal reamers.
4. *Acute respiratory infection* is an absolute contraindication to general anaesthesia, as broncho-pneumonia may follow.
5. *Chronic respiratory disease* may require elimination of dental sepsis in an effort to prevent inhalation of infected material from the mouth.
6. *Pulmonary TB* cases who are not declared safe should be barrier treated and care must be taken to ensure proper sterilisation of all instruments used.

Haematology

ANAEMIA

A common and important condition which may produce the
following clinical features:
1. Pallor (best seen in the mucosal surfaces)
2. Fatigue and lassitude
3. Breathlessness on exertion
4. Tachycardia and palpitations
5. Smooth sore tongue

CAUSES OF ANAEMIA

(A) Deficient r.b.c. production
1. *Deficiency* of
   Fe
   B_{12} or folic acid
   Vitamin C
   Protein
2. *Aplastic anaemia*
3. *Marrow infiltration*
   Leukaemia
   Lymphoma, e.g. Hodgkin's
   Myeloma
   Myelosclerosis
   Metastatic carcinoma
4. *'Symptomatic'*
   Anaemia of chronic infection
   Uraemia
   Liver disease
   Malignancy
   Collagen-vascular disease, e.g. SLE, Rheumatoid disease

(B) Loss or destruction of r.b.c.s
1. *Haemorrhage*
2. *Haemolysis*
3. *Hypersplenism*

Some RBC abnormalities seen in a blood film

Size
Anisocytosis — variation in size, due to anaemia
Macrocytosis — seen in a film as increased diameter of r.b.c.'s, but
   defined as an increase in mean corpuscular *volume*
Microcytosis — defined as a decrease in mean corpuscular *volume*

Shape
Poikilocytosis — variation in shape, due to anaemia which is
   usually severe
Spherocytosis — spheroidal cells seen in hereditary spherocytosis
   and in acquired haemolytic anaemia
Elliptocytosis — elliptical cells. Hereditary. Haemolytic anaemia
   may or may not occur
Sickling — crescentic cells seen when reducing agents act on Hb S.
   Hereditary. Sickle-cell anaemia may or may not occur
Bizarre shapes — seen in severe uraemia and carcinomatosis

Staining
Hypochromia — decreased intensity of stain, due to Fe deficiency
Polychromasia — diffuse basophilia. Indicates active blood
   regeneration, just as reticulocytosis does
Punctate basophilia — stippled appearance seen in severe anaemia
   or lead poisoning
Target cells (Mexican hat cells) occur in:
   (i) Fe deficiency
   (ii) liver disease
   (iii) after splenectomy

Causes of haemolytic anaemia

(*A*) *Congenital*
1. Spherocytosis ('acholuric jaundice')
2. Haemoglobinopathy
   (i) sickle-cell anaemia
   (ii) thalassaemia syndromes
3. Non-spherocytic (enzyme defects)

(*B*) *Acquired*
1. Auto-immune haemolysins
   (i) Idiopathic warm or cold antibodies
   (ii) Viral or mycoplasmal infection
2. Secondary (symptomatic)
   (i) Chronic lymphatic leukaemia
   (ii) Malignant lymphoma
   (iii) SLE
   (iv) Malaria

(v) Uncommonly —
renal disease
liver disease
carcinoma
rheumatoid disease
TB or syphilis
3. Drugs and chemicals, e.g. lead, methyldopa
4. Haemolytic disease of the newborn

Macrocytic anaemia

Causes of folic acid deficiency
1. Dietary deficiency or malabsorption
2. Pregnancy
3. Increased cell turnover, e.g. leukaemia or reticulosis
4. Anti-folate drugs, e.g. anticonvulsants

Causes of vitamin B_{12} deficiency
1. Pernicious anaemia or gastrectomy
2. Changed intestinal flora, e.g. blind-loop syndrome
3. Ileal disease, e.g. Crohn's

Clinical features of Addisonian pernicious anaemia
1. Usually over 30, may have blue eyes, fair hair, premature greying
2. Anaemia of insidious onset
3. Glossitis, often intermittent
4. GI symptoms, e.g. dyspepsia, diarrhoea
5. Subacute combined degeneration
   (i) Peripheral neuritis
   (ii) Dorso-lateral column involvement
   (iii) Mental changes
   (iv) Rarely optic atrophy, nystagmus, impotence, etc.
        N.B. may be mixed upper motor-neurone and lower motor-neurone signs
6. Mild pyrexia
7. Slight hepato-splenomegaly
8. Retinal haemorrhage
9. Increased incidence of Ca stomach

Causes of pancytopenia
1. Aplastic anaemia (q.v.)
2. Acute leukaemia (in subleukaemic phase)
3. Marrow infiltration:
   (i) Malignant lymphoma
   (ii) Metastatic carcinoma
   (iii) Myelomatosis
   (iv) Myelosclerosis (in late stages)

4. Hypersplenism
5. Pernicious anaemia
6. SLE
7. Rarely, disseminated TB

Causes of neutropenia severe enough to cause symptoms (agranulocytosis)
1. Aplastic anaemia
   (i) Idiopathic
   (ii) Drugs, e.g.
       cytotoxic drugs
       phenylbutazone
       chloramphenicol
   (iii) Chemicals, e.g. benzene
   (iv) Radiation
2. Selective drug-induced neutropenia (normal Hb and platelets)
3. Acute leukaemia (in subleukaemic phase)
4. Hypersplenism
5. Idiopathic (rare)

POLYCYTHAEMIA
Polycythaemia is increased mass of red cells in the blood, as estimated by the haematocrit.
1. *Compensatory* — to increase oxygen-carrying capacity of blood, in
   (a) Chronic respiratory disease e.g. emphysema (poor oxygenation of blood)
   (b) Congenital heart disease — especially with an a-v shunt (inadequate oxygenation of tissues)
   (c) High altitudes — where there is reduced oxygen in inspired air
2. *Polycythaemia rubra vera*
An uncommon condition of unknown aetiology. Marrow hyperplasia produces increased number of red cells. The skin has a dusky purple colouration due to red cell congestion of blood vessels. There may also be vertigo, tinnitus, visual disturbances and headache, for the same reason. There is a tendency to thrombosis.

Causes of neutrophil leucocytosis
1. Bacterial infections
2. Myeloproliferative disease
   Myeloid leukaemia
   Myelosclerosis
   Polycythaemia vera
3. Haemorrhage, especially internal

4. Tissue damage
   Trauma (including surgery)
   Burns
   Myocardial infarction
5. Malignancy, especially necrotic tumours and hepatic metastases
6. Drugs, especially steroids

Causes of eosinophilia
1. *Allergy*
   Hypersensitivity to food or drugs
2. *Parasites*
   e.g. trichiniasis, hydatid
3. *Skin disease*
   (i) Scabies
   (ii) Atopy (eczema, urticaria, hay fever, asthma)
   (iii) Dermatitis herpetiformis
4. *Pulmonary eosinophilia*
A range of disease characterized by radiographic pulmonary
infiltrates, eosiniphilia, and varying degrees of asthma and
vasculitis, e.g. Löffler's disease and the pulmonary form of
polyarteritis nodosa
5. *Malignancy*, especially Hodgkin's disease

Causes of polycythaemia
1. Polycythaemia vera
2. Hypoxia, e.g.
   (i) High altitude
   (ii) Cyanotic heart disease
   (iii) Pulmonary disease
   (iv) Obesity
3. Miscellaneous causes of increased erythropoietin, e.g.
   (i) Kidney cyst, neoplasm or hydronephrosis
   (ii) Liver carcinoma
   (iii) Cerebellar haemangioblastoma

Clinical features of polycythaemia vera
1. Headache, dizziness and lassitude
2. Plethoric appearance: engorged conjunctival and retinal
   vessels
3. Hypertension
4. Splenomegaly
5. Generalized pruritus
6. Dyspepsia due to GI vessel enlargement, or associated peptic
   ulcer
7. Thrombosis, e.g. cerebral, coronary or mesenteric
8. Haemorrhagic tendency
9. Peripheral ischaemia due to slow circulation or thrombosis
10. Gout

Causes of splenomegaly
1. *Infections* especially infectious mononucleosis, septicaemia, bacterial endocarditis and malaria
2. *Blood dyscrasis*
    (i) Leukaemia (especially chronic myeloid)
    (ii) Haemolytic anaemia
    (iii) Myelosclerosis
    (iv) Polycythaemia vera
3. *Malignant lymphomas*
4. *Portal hypertension*
5. *Lipoid storage disease*
6. *Occasionally in rheumatoid disease and SLE*

Causes of lymphadenopathy
1. *Infections*
    (i) Focal infection with regional lymphadenopathy, e.g. sepsis, TB, primary chancre
    (ii) Infectious mononucleosis
    (iii) Rubella
    (iv) Secondary syphilis
    (v) Toxoplasmosis
    (vi) Tropical infestation, e.g. filariasis
2. *Lymphoma*
    (i) Hodgkin's
    (ii) Non-Hodgkin's
        (a) Follicular
        (b) Diffuse
3. *Leukaemia*, usually lymphatic
4. *Malignancy*
    (i) Metastases
    (ii) Reactive changes
5. *Miscellaneous*
    (i) Sarcoidosis
    (ii) Histiocytosis X
    (iii) Chronic inflammatory skin disease
    (iv) Collagen vascular disease, e.g. RA, SLE
    (v) Anticonvulsant drugs

CLINICAL FEATURES OF HODGKIN'S DISEASE
1. Weight loss, malaise, lassitude
2. Fever (the periodic Pel-Ebstein pattern is uncommon)
3. Large, discrete, rubbery superficial lymph nodes
4. Mediastinal or retroperitoneal node involvement
5. Hepato-splenomegaly
6. Pulmonary or pleural infiltration
7. Pain or paralysis due to pressure on nerves or spinal cord
8. Marrow infiltration with pain or pathological fracture

9. Skin
   pruritus
   pigmentation
   herpes zoster
   nodular infiltrates
10. Infections due to decreased cell-mediated immunity
11. Alcohol-induced pain

CLINICAL FEATURES OF THE THREE COMMON LEUKAEMIAS

Anaemia, constitutional symptons (fever, malaise, weight loss) and bleeding (including purpura) occur in all three types but are more severe in acute leukaemia and less severe in chronic lymphatic leukaemia

Acute leukaemia
1. Occurs at any age
2. Onset may be abrupt or insidious
3. Stomatitis and pharyngitis
4. Susceptibility to infections, especially of upper respiratory tract
5. Slight lymphadenopathy
6. Slight or moderate liver and spleen enlargement
7. Bone and joint pain, with sternal tenderness

Chronic lymphatic leukaemia
1. Occurs in late middle age, more often in males
2. Insidious onset, often found accidentally
3. Moderate or marked lymphadenopathy
4. Recurrent chronic infections
5. Moderate liver and spleen enlargement
6. May be haemolytic anaemia
7. Skin lesions
   pruritus
   herpes zoster
   nodular infiltrates
   l'homme rough

CLINICAL FEATURES OF MYELOMATOSIS
1. Progressive anaemia
2. Bone pain
   (i) osteolytic lesions
   (ii) pathological fractures
   (iii) osteomalacia (due to renal phosphate leak)
3. Bleeding, due to thrombocytopenia
4. Fever

5. Renal involvement
   (i) acute or chronic uraemia
   (ii) Fanconi syndrome (failure of tubular reabsorption)
6. Hepatomegaly, occasionally with jaundice
7. Hypercalcaemia
8. Hyperuricaemia
9. Amyloidosis
10. Neuropathy, with raised c.s.f. protein
11. Susceptibility to infections, due to defective antibodies

BLEEDING

May be due to defects of platelets, coagulation or vessels

Causes of thrombocytopenia
1. Idiopathic thrombocytopenic purpura
2. Causes of pancytopenia
3. Drugs causing selective thrombocytopenia, e.g. salicylates
4. Incompatible or massive blood transfusions
N.B. In thrombocytopenia, bleeding time and capillary fragility are increased, but coagulation time is *normal*

Coagulation disorders

1. Congenital
(a) Haemophilias
   (i) Haemophilia A (VIII deficiency)
   (ii) Haemophilia B (IX deficiency, Christmas disease)
   (iii) von Willebrand's disease (vascular defect + VIII deficiency)
(b) Other congenital deficiencies
   Factors I, II, V, VII, X, XI, XII or XIII

2. Acquired
   (i) Vitamin K deficiency
   (ii) Liver disease
   (iii) Anticoagulant drugs
   (iv) Defibrination syndrome (consumption coagulopathy)
   (v) Acute primary fibrinolysis
   (vi) Massive transfusion of stored blood
   (vii) Circulating inhibitors of coagulation

Causes of bleeding due to small vessel defects

Congenital
1. Hereditary haemorrhagic telangiectasia (Osler–Weber–Rendu)
2. Von Willebrand's disease
3. Pseudo-xanthoma elasticum

Acquired
1. *Infection* e.g. Bacterial endocarditis, septicaemia, especially meningococcal
2. *Drugs* e.g. Corticosteriods, carbromal
3. *Secondary to systemic disease* ('*symptomatic*')
    (i) Cushing's
    (ii) Scurvy
    (iii) Dysproteinaemia
    (iv) Polyarteritis nodosa
4. '*Allergic*' *vasculitis*
    (i) Henoch–Schönlein purpura
    (ii) Cutaneous vasculitis
5. *Miscellaneous*
    (i) Simple easy bruising
    (ii) Senile purpura
    (iii) Dermatoses, e.g. eczema
    (iv) Fat embolism

BLOOD DISEASES AND THE DENTAL SURGEON

Almost all blood disorders are of importance to the dental surgeon.

1. Haemorrhagic diatheses

Obviously important where dental procedures produce bleeding. These patients should be thoroughly investigated by a haematologist prior to treatment. In such cases local analgesic injections may cause profuse bleeding, so until advised differently by a haematologist all potentially harmful treatment should be withheld.
Any case of prolonged post-extraction haemorrhage should be thoroughly investigated by a haematologist as there may be an underlying predisposition to haemorrhage such as a vessel, platelet or coagulation defect.

2. Anaemia

This common disorder with its oral symptoms makes any complaint of a sore tongue an indication for blood examination. Anaemic patients do not withstand blood loss well. Further blood loss in an already anaemic patient may provoke heart failure or myocardial infarction. Multiple extractions should be postponed until the anaemia is corrected.

3. Leukaemia

Often the earliest signs of this disease are gingival bleeding or soreness or ulceration. The responsibilities of the dentist in recognizing and referring for early diagnosis of this serious condition are obvious. Operative dental procedures for these patients may lead to prolonged bleeding or severe sepsis. Consultation with the patient's physician is mandatory.

Endocrinology

THE PITUITARY

This consists of an anterior lobe derived from the embryonic mouth and a posterior lobe which is a downward extension of the brain. The anterior part produces secretions which control all other endocrine glands.

Hypothalamic control of the anterior pituitary

Stimulating hormones
1. Thyrotrophin releasing factor (TRF)
2. Corticotrophin releasing factor (CRF)
3. Somatotrophin (GH) releasing factor (SRF)
4. Luteinising hormone releasing factor (LRF)
5. Follicle-stimulating hormone releasing factor (FRF)

Inhibiting hormones
1. Prolactin inhibiting factor (PIF)
2. Melanocyte-stimulating hormone inhibiting factor (MIF)

Clinical features of acromegaly   HYPERPITUITARISM

Symptoms   EXS Growth hormone after
1. Often insidious, with no symptoms   epyphyses have
2. Headaches
3. Paraesthesiae (median nerve compression)   closed
4. Weakness and joint pains
5. Visual deterioration.   otherwise gigantism

Signs

1. Characteristics facies, large hands and feet
2. Leathery furrowed skin. May be seborrhoea, hyperhidrosis or pigmentation
3. Hoarse deep voice
4. Nontoxic goitre

5. Progressive kyphosis
6. Bitemporal hemianopia, optic atrophy, ocular palsies
7. Generalized splanchnomegaly
8. Cardiac failure (hypertension and ischaemia)
9. Signs of diabetes mellitus or its complications
10. Hypopituitarism

Causes of hypopituitarism
1. Tumours
   Eosinophil adenoma, chromophobe adenoma, etc.
2. Iatrogenic — hypophysectomy or irradiation
3. Pituitary necrosis due to ante- or post-partum haemorrhage
   (Sheehan's syndrome)
4. Granulomatous infiltration, eg sarcoidosis
5. Trauma
6. Infection, eg TB meningitis

Clinical features of hypopituitarism
Loss of anterior pituitary hormones is usually partial, in the
following order of frequency.
1. *Somatotrophin (GH)*
   Dwarfism in children
   Insulin sensitivity in adults
2. *Prolactin*
   Failure of lactation in post-partum patients
3. *Gonadotrophins*
   Delayed puberty in children
   Loss of body hair, fine wrinkled skin, impotence, infertility and
   amenorrhoea in adults
4. *Thyrotrophin (TSH)*
   Hypothyroidism
5. *Corticotrophin (ACTH)*
   Hypoadrenalism (asthenia, nausea, vomiting, hypoglycaemia,
   collapse)
6. *Melanocyte-stimulating hormone (MSH)*
   Skin pallor

Clinical features of hypothalamic lesions
1. Diabetes insipidus with variable deficiencies of anterior pituitary
   hormones
2. Obesity
3. Somnolence
4. Variations in body temperature
5. Precocious puberty
6. Irregular menstruation

THE THYROID

Causes of hypothyroidism

(A) Primary (Thyroid gland failure)
1. Autoimmune thyroiditis
   Hashimoto's disease and its atrophic variant, myxoedema. In Hashimoto's the thyroid is large and may be tender, but in myxoedema it is impalpable. Circulating thyroid antibodies occur in both.
2. Iatrogenic
   Surgery
   Irradiation
   Antithyroid drugs
3. Endemic cretinism (maternal iodine deficiency)

(B) Secondary (TSH deficiency)
1. Pituitary lesion
2. Rarely hypothalamic lesion (due to thyrotrophin releasing factor deficiency)

Clinical features of hypothyroidism
1. Mental and physical sluggishness
2. Cold intolerance
3. Constipation
4. Weight gain
5. Croaking voice, with slow speech
6. Rough, dry yellowish skin
7. 'Myxoedema facies' with generalized thickening of subcutaneous tissue, periorbital puffiness, brittle sparse hair and thin eyebrows.
8. Bradycardia
9. Delayed relaxation of tendon jerks
Less commonly —
10. Anaemia or angina
11. Carpal tunnel syndrome
12. Perceptive deafness
13. Myalgia or arthralgia
14. 'Myxoedema madness' (rare)
15. Coma (rare)

Causes of 'non-toxic' goitre
1. 'Simple' colloid goitre (idiopathic), common during puberty and pregnancy
2. Iodine deficiency
3. Goitrogens, e.g. antithyroid drugs, excess iodine
4. Auto-immune thyroiditis (Hashimoto's)

Possibility of malignancy is suggested by:
1. Asymmetrical enlargement with 'cold area' on scan
2. Very hard thyroid
3. Pressure effects, e.g. hoarseness
4. Cervical lymphadenopathy

Causes of hyperthyroidism
1. Graves' disease
2. Toxic multinodular goitre. Resembles Graves' disease but patients tend to be older, with fewer eye signs
3. Toxic adenoma
4. Iatrogenic (excess thyroid hormone)

Clinical features of Graves' disease

Thyroid gland
1. Goitre, usually diffuse (but may be nodular)
2. Increased thyroid vascularity (thrill, bruit)

Metabolic
3. Increased heat production (warm moist skin, heat intolerance)
4. Weight loss, increased appetite, diarrhoea
5. Tachycardia, exertional dyspnoea, hyperdynamic circulation
6. Tiredness, irritability, nervousness
7. Fine tremor, hyperkinesia
8. Proximal muscle weakness with hyperactive reflexes
9. In elderly patients, atrial fibrillation or cardiac failure
10. Eye signs
    Eyelid oedema
    Conjunctivitis
    Exophthalmos
    Lid retraction or lag
    Ophthalmoplegia (usually superior rectus)

Management of thyrotoxicosis
1. *Indications for thyroidectomy*
    (i) Possible malignancy
    (ii) Pressure symptoms
    (iii) Retrosternal goitre
    (iv) Large goitre
    (v) Refusal or failure of medical treatment
    (vi) Hypersensitivity to antithyroid drugs
2. *Indications for medical treatment*
    (i) Children
    (iii) Pregnancy
    (iii) Mild hyperthyroidism with small goitre
    (iv) Patients unsuitable for surgery

3. *Indications for radio-iodine therapy*
    (i) Relapse after thyroidectomy
    (ii) Patients over age 45
    Subsequent hypothyroidism is common (about 40% at 10 years)

THE PARATHYROIDS

Causes of hyperparathyroidism
1. *Primary*
Adenoma (85%)
Hyperplasia
Carcinoma
2. *Secondary*
Hyperplasia due to chronic renal failure, osteomalacia or rickets

Clinical features of hyperparathyroidism
1. *Due to hypercalcaemia*
    (i) Anorexia, nausea and vomiting
    (ii) Constipation
    (iii) Polydipsia and polyuria
    (iv) Lethargy progressing to coma and convulsions
2. *Metastatic calcification*
    (i) Renal calculi
    (ii) Nephrocalcinosis
    (iii) Conjunctival deposits and keratopathy
3. *Bone resorption*
    (i) Pain and deformity
    (ii) Pathological fractures

Causes of hypoparathyroidism
1. Post-operative (e.g. thyroidectomy)
2. Idiopathic (possibly autoimmune)
3. Neonatal (transient, but dangerous)

Clinical features of hypoparathyroidism
1. *Due to hypocalcaemia*
    (i) Tetany (paraesthesiae, stridor, cramps, hyperreflexia)
        Trousseau's and Chvostek's signs are present
    (ii) Convulsions (especially in children)
    (iii) Cataracts
2. *In idiopathic hypoparathyroidism*
    (i) Mental subnormality
    (ii) Dry skin, sparse hair, poor teeth, nail dystrophy often with
        candidosis
    (iii) Papilloedema and calcified basal ganglia (mimics brain
        tumour)

(iv) Other auto-immune disorders, e.g.
      hypoadrenalism
      pernicious anaemia

CUSHING'S SYNDROME   ADRENAL HYPERSECRETION

Clinical features
1. Obesity of trunk and face with 'buffalo hump'
2. Hypertension
3. Skin changes
      Striae
      Bruising
      Hirsutism
      Pigmentation
4. Osteoporosis
5. Proximal myopathy
6. Menstrual disturbances
7. Neurosis or psychosis
8. Facial plethora due to polycythaemia

Laboratory features
1. Increased plasm 11-hydroxycorticosteroids ('cortisol')
      Normal values —

9 a.m.	12 midnight
190–690 mmol/1	80–190 nmol/l
(7–25 µg/100 ml)	(3–7 µg/100 ml)

      Loss of diurnal rhythm occurs early in Cushing's syndrome
      (i.e. midnight samples give increased value)
2. Polycythaemia with leucocytosis and eosinophil decrease
3. Hypokalaemia, with sodium in upper normal range
4. 'Diabetic' glucose tolerance test
5. 24 hour urinary 'free 11-hydroxycorticosteroids' increased
Low dosage dexamethasone (0.5 mg q.d.s. for 2 days) causes little suppression in Cushing's syndrome
High dosage dexamathasone (2 mg q.d.s. for 2 days) causes suppression in adrenal hyperplasia, but has little or no effect in adrenal adenoma or carcinoma, or ectopic ACTH secretion due to extra-adrenal carcinoma.

CAUSES OF HYPOADRENALISM

Acute
1. Stress occurring in patients with chronic hypoadrenalism
2. Septicaemia, especially meningococcal
3. Surgical adrenalectomy, e.g. for breast cancer

Chronic

(A) Primary
1. Auto-immune adrenalitis (Addison's)
2. TB
3. Metastatic cancer deposits occur commonly, but rarely cause hypoadrenalism

(B) Secondary (ACTH deficiency)
1. Pituitary or hypothalamic disease
2. Prolonged corticosteroid therapy

Clinical features of chronic hypoadrenalism
1. Pigmentation, especially in exposed skin, mouth, areolae, palmar creases and pressure areas
2. Debility and tiredness
3. Nausea, vomiting, weight loss, abdnominal pain, diarrhoea
4. Hypotension, with low-income pulse
5. Hypoglycaemia, especially reactive after a meal
6. Loss of body hair in women
7. Depression

Laboratory features of hypoadrenalism
1. Plasma 11-hydroxycorticosteroids may be normal or low, but fail to respond adequately to 250 μg Synacthen® IM (should rise by more than 193 nmol/l (7 μg/100 ml) at 30 minutes)
2. Slow excretion of a water load
3. Low plasma sodium and chloride, with raised potassium and urea.
4. Low voltage ECG with flat T waves
5. Low blood sugar

DIABETES MELLITUS

Differences between the two main types of diabetes mellitus

Juvenile	Maturity onset
1. Thin	Obese
2. Young	Middle-aged or elderly
3. Tendency to ketosis	Resistant to ketosis
4. Low insulin secretion	Normal or increased insulin secretion
5. Sensitive to insulin	Insulin resistant
Require treatment with insulin	Respond to diet and oral hypoglycaemic drugs

Differences between 'diabetic' and hypoglycaemic coma

Ketoacidaemic coma	Hypoglycaemic coma
1. Preceded by infection or insulin underdosage	Preceded by exercise, missed meal or insulin overdosage
2. Onset over hours or days	Onset in minutes
3. Deep rapid breathing	Stertorous breathing
4. Dehydration	Normal hydration
5. Sweating absent	Sweating marked
6. CNS changes unusual	CNS changes common, especially Babinski response
7. Urine — usually glycosuria and ketonuria	Urine not helpful

Complications of diabetes mellitus

1. Ocular
  (i) Blurred vision due to fluctuations in blood sugar
 (ii) Cataracts
(iii) Retinopathy
       Venous engorgement
       Capillary microaneurysms
       'Blot' haemorrhages
       'Waxy' exudates
       Retinitis proliferans
       Retinal detachment
       Vitreous haemorrhage and fibrosis
(iv) Rubeosis iridis (new blood vessels over iris) — may cause
       glaucoma

2. Neurological
  (i) Peripheral neuropathy (early sign is loss of ankle jerks and
       malleolar vibration sense)
 (ii) Mononeuritis multiplex (neuropathy of several peripheral or
       cranial nerves; often asymmetrical)
(iii) Autonomic neuropathy
       diarrhoea
       postural hypotension
       impotence
       abnormal sweating
       dependent oedema

3. Renal
   (i) Pyelonephritis, sometimes with papillary necrosis
  (ii) Glomerulonephritis
       (a) Kimmelstiel-Wilson (eosinophilic nodules in glomerular tuft)
       (b) Proliferative, with sclerosed basement membrane
 (iii) Atherosclerosis and hypertensive vascular changes

4. Vascular
Occlusion by atheroma (large vessels) or endarteritis (small vessels) may cause ischaemia of feet, myocardium, brain or kidneys.

5. Dermatological
   (i) Fat atrophy or hypertrophy at insulin injection sites
  (ii) Ulcers due to neuropathy or ischaemia
 (iii) Infections, especially furuncles and candidosis
 (iv) Pigmented scars over shins ('diabetic dermopathy')
  (v) Xanthomata
 (vi) Necrobiosis lipoidica

6. Systemic infections
Incidence of TB and deep mycoses is increased

CAUSES OF DWARFISM

1. *'Consitutional'*
   Racial, familial or sporadic
2. *Nutritional*
   (i) Starvation
  (ii) Malabsorption
 (iii) Protein loss
3. *Chromosomal defects*
   (i) Trisomies, e.g. Down's
  (ii) Turner's
4. *Skeletal defects*
   (i) Rickets
   (i) Achondroplasia
 (iii) Gargoylism (Hurler's)
5. *Chronic systemic disease*
   (i) Cyanotic congenital heart disease
  (ii) Renal failure
 (iii) Hepatic failure
 (iv) Pulmonary disease
  (v) Anaemia
 (vi) Infections, e.g. TB

6. *Endocrine disease*
    (i) Sexual precocity
    (ii) Hypopituitarism
    (iii) Hypothyroidism
    (iv) Congenital adrenal hyperplasia

CAUSES OF HIRSUTISM

1. 'Constitutional' (often racial or familial)
2. Stein-Leventhal syndrome (polycystic ovaries)
3. Virilizing ovarian tumours, e.g. arrhenoblastoma
4. Cushing's syndrome
5. Congenital adrenal hyperplasia (of late onset)
6. Adrenal tumours

OSTEOPOROSIS

A reduction in bone mass below the normal expected for the age and sex of the patient. Histologically the trabecular bone is reduced, and the mineral-matrix ration is approximately normal.

Common causes
1. Old age
2. Immobilization
3. Glucocorticoid therapy (or Cushing's disease)
4. Rheumatoid arthritis causes localized osteoporosis

OSTEOMALACIA

A reduction in the mineral-matrix ratio, although the total bone mass may be normal, decreased or even increased.

Common causes
1. Deficiency of cholecalciferol (vitamin D)
    (i) Inadequate diet, possibly aggravated by pregnancy or lack of UV radiation
    (ii) Malabsorption
2. Chronic renal failure

ENDOCRINE DISEASES IN RELATION TO DENTISTRY

Many endocrine disorders show characteristic features which effect the face and oral cavity, so dental surgeons have a special responsibility for recognizing these signs and referring the patient for medical assessment.
Thyrotoxicosis and diabetes mellitus are by far the most common conditions and therefore more likely to be encountered.

Acromegaly causes continued growth particularly of the mandible and tongue. This leads to prognathism and spacing of the teeth.

In Addison's disease there may be brown pigmentation of the oral mucosa.

Poorly-controlled diabetics are very prone to gingival disease and periodontal abscesses. Prior to general anaesthesia diabetics require careful regulation of their carbohydrates and insulin regimes. They should not be allowed to become hypoglycaemic during dental treatment.

Patients with thyrotoxicosis are frequently recognizable by their exophthalmos and require careful management due to their anxious and excitable state. Many authorities recommend adrenaline-free local anaesthetics as these patients are very prone to tachycardia. General anaesthesia requires expert administration.

Cretinism is a rare condition and causes delayed bone development as well as delayed eruption of teeth.

Hyperparathyroidism causes areas of resorption in bones, including the mandible.

Gastro-intestinal system

Causes of atrophic glossitis (*smooth red tongue*)
1. Antibiotics
2. Anaemia due to deficiency of Fe, B_{12} or folate
3. Vitamin deficiency (riboflavin or nicotinic acid)

Common causes of severe upper GI bleeding
1. Duodenal ulcer
2. Oesophageal varices
3. Erosive gastritis
4. Gastric ulcer
5. Erosive oesophagitis

Common causes of severe lower GI bleeding
1. Ulcerative colitis
2. Carcinoma of rectum or colon
3. Benign rectal polyps
4. Haemorrhoids or anal fissure
5. Rectal trauma, including biopsy

CAUSES OF DYSPHAGIA

1. Lesions of mouth or pharynx
     (i) Stomatitis or glossitis
    (ii) Tonsillitis
   (iii) Quinsy, retropharyngeal abscess
    (iv) Lymphoma of tonsil
2. Foreign body in pharynx or oesophagus
3. Intrinsic disease of pharynx or oesophagus
     (i) Plummer-Vinson syndrome — iron deficiency, glossitis, pharyngeal web and koilonychia
    (ii) Pharyngeal pouch
   (iii) Inflammation, stricture or neoplasm of oesophagus
    (iv) Systemic sclerosis
     (v) Oesophageal achalasia

4. Extrinsic compression
  (i) Tumours in neck
  (ii) Mediastinal tumour, e.g. retrosternal goitre, lymph nodes
  (iii) Bronchial cancer
  (iv) Aortic aneurysm
5. CNS lesions
  (i) Bulbar or pseudo-bulbar palsy
  (i) Myasthenia gravis
  (iii) Congenital muscular incoordination

PEPTIC ULCERS

Table 1. Differences between gastric and duodenal ulcers

	Gastric	Duodenal
Site	Usually middle 2/3 of lesser curve	Usually duodenal bulb
Gastric acid	Low or normal	Hyperchlorhydria
Pain	After meals	Relieved by meals May occur at about 2 a.m.
Vomiting	Common	Uncommon
Sex	Equal prevalence	4 × as common in men
Social class	Commoner in lower social classes	Equal prevalence
Pathology	May be benign or malignant	Virtually never malignant

Factors suggesting a gastric ulcer is malignant

Symptoms
1. Anorexia and weight loss
2. Epigastric pain not related to food
3. Dysphagia

Signs
1. Epigastric mass
2. Metastases. Look especially for
  (i) Large irregular liver
  (ii) Supraclavicular nodes
  (iii) Deep vein thrombosis of leg
  (iv) Ascites

Barium meal
1. Filling defect and failure of peristalsis in a site other than middle 2/3 of lesser curve
2. Very large ulcer anywhere in the stomach
3. Leather-bottle stomach
If in doubt gastroscopy and gastric cytology may help

Complications of peptic ulcer
1. Bleeding
2. Penetration, e.g. into pancreas, liver or retroperitoneal space
3. Perforation
4. Obstruction
   (i) Oedema and spasm — reversible
   (ii) Cicatricial stenosis — irreversible
5. 'Milk-alkali syndrome' — alkalosis and calcinosis, due to excessive ingestion of milk, alkali and calcium salts.

CAUSES OF MALABSORPTION

1. Inadequate digestion
   (i) Gastric or intestinal resection
   (ii) Hepatic or biliary tract obstruction
   (iii) Pancreatic insufficiency (especially fibrocystic disease)
2. Parasites or change in intestinal flora
   (i) Tape worms
   (ii) Blind-loop syndromes (after intestinal surgery)
3. Intestinal hurry or fistulae
4. Coeliac syndrome
5. Tropical sprue
6. Intestinal infiltration
   (i) TB
   (ii) Lymphoma, leukaemia
7. Enzyme defects (e.g. Disaccharidase deficiency)
8. Chronic intestinal ischaemia (e.g. atheroma)

Clinical features of idopathic steatorrhoea (adult coeliac syndrome)
1. Loose stools which may or may not be bulky, pale and foul-smelling
2. Weight loss (fat and protein deficiency)
3. Oedema (protein deficiency)
4. Flatulence with distended abdomen (impaired disaccharide hydrolysis)
5. Hypochromic anaemia (Fe deficiency)
6. Macrocytic anaemic (folate or B_{12} deficiency)
7. Peripheral neuritis (B-complex deficiency)
8. Glossitis and stomatitis (B-complex deficiency)
9. Osteomalacia (Ca and vitamin D deficiency)

10. Paraesthesiae, tetany (Ca or Mg deficiency)
11. Haemorrhage (vitamin K deficiency)
12. Muscle flaccidity, arrhythmias (potassium deficiency)
13. Weakness and hypotension (water and electrolyte deficiency)
14. Clubbing

CAUSES OF ASCITES

1. Carcinoma, especially ovarian or alimentary
2. Cirrhosis
3. Hypoalbuminaemia, e.g. nephrotic syndrome
4. Constrictive pericarditis, congestive heart failure
5. Thrombosis or obstruction of inferior vena cava

CAUSES OF OBSTRUCTION OF THE SMALL INTESTINE

The commonest causes are adhesions secondary to operation and bowel incarceration in an internal or external hernia.

(A) Mechanical
1. Compression from without:
   Adhesions
   Fibrous bands
   Tumours, especially of female pelvic organs
2. Hernia
3. Strictures
   Congenital atresia
   Acquired
   Inflammatory
   Neoplastic
   Traumatic
4. Obturation
   Gallstones
   Faecal impaction
   Meconium ileus (in babies)
5. Volvulus
6. Intussusception

(B) Paralytic ileus
1. Abdminal surgery
2. Peritonitis
3. Acute systemic illness, e.g. pneumonia
4. Painful lumbar conditions, e.g. renal colic,
5. Mesenteric ischaemia
6. Drugs, e.g. ganglion-blockers
7. Hypokalaemia

ACUTE ABDOMINAL PAIN

Two main causes of this symptom are:
1. *Smooth muscle spasm.* Follows obstruction of the lumen of a hollow viscus, e.g. acute intestinal obstruction (intestinal colic), biliary colic or ureteric ('renal') colic.
2. *Inflammation of a viscus.* This causes peritoneal inflammation and pain, e.g. perforation of a peptic ulcer, acute appendicitis, acute cholecystitis. In peritoneal inflammation the abdominal wall muscles adopt a board-like rigidity.

MEDICAL CAUSES OF ACUTE ABDOMINAL PAIN

Common causes
1. Food poisoning or dietary indiscretion
2. Peptic ulcer, gastritis, oesophagitis
3. Biliary colic or cholecystitis
4. Pancreatitis
5. Hepatic congestion (hepatitis, cardiac failure)
6. Renal colic, pyelonephritis or cystitis
7. Diverticulitis, ulcerative colitis, regional ileitis
8. Mesenteric adenitis (children)
9. Mesenteric ischaemia (atheroma, embolism, polyarteritis nodosa)
10. Aortic dissection
11. Gynaecological, e.g.
    Mittlelschmerz (ovulation)
    Dysmenorrhoea
    Salpingitis
    Threatened abortion
12. Pain referred from spine or chest

N.B. Pain in the abdomen which lasts for more than 6 hours without remission is likely to be surgical.

CAUSES OF HEPATOMEGALY

1. Hepatic congestion, e.g. cardiac failure hepatic vein thrombosis
2. Neoplasm
    (i) Metastases
    (ii) Lymphoma
    (iii) Hepatoma
3. Myeloproliferative disease, e.g. leukaemia, myelofibrosis
4. Infective
    (i) Viral, e.g. hepatitis
    (ii) Bacterial, e.g. Weil's disease
    (iii) Protozoal, e.g. amoebic abscess
    (iv) Parasitic, e.g. hydatid cyst

5. Biliary obstruction
6. Fatty infiltration or early cirrhosis
7. Storage disorders, e.g. amyloidosis

REGIONAL ILEITIS (CROHN'S DISEASE)

Clinical features
1. Usually young adults
2. Malaise, weakness, weight loss, pyrexia
3. Intermittent colicky pain in R. iliac fossa
4. Mild or moderate diarrhoea
5. Tenderness in R. iliac fossa, sometimes with a fixed mass

Complications
1. Obstruction due to stricture
2. Perforation
3. Abscess
4. Fistula into anus, bladder or abdominal wall
5. Fissure-in-ano
6. Malabsorption (especially B_{12})
7. Procto-colitis
8. Erythema nodosum
9. Clubbing

Ba studies (may need both meal and enema)
1. Luminal narrowing of ileum (Kantor's 'string sign')
2. Distorted mucosal pattern
3. 'Skip' lesions
The correlation between radiological appearance and disease
activity is often poor.

DIVERTICULITIS

Clinical features
1. Usually middle-aged or elderly
2. Recurrent bouts of colicky abdominal pain
3. Nausea and vomiting
4. May be either constipation or diarrhoea
5. Tenderness in L. iliac fassa, sometimes with a mass

Complications
1. Obstruction due to stricture
2. Perforation
3. Abscess
4. Fistula into bladder or vagina

Ba enema
1. Diverticula may or may not be seen
2. Segmental spasm and irritability of the affected colon (usually sigmoid)
3. Chronic fibrotic deformity

ULCERATIVE COLITIS

Clinical features
1. Commonly presents in 3rd or 4th decade
2. Malaise, weakness, weight loss, pyrexia
3. Chronic diarrhoea, with blood and mucus, which is often severe
4. Pain in L. iliac fossa, and rectal tenesmus

Complications
1. Perforation
2. Perianal abscess
3. Acute 'toxic dilatation'
4. Severe haemorrhage
5. Hypokalaemia, hypoproteinaemia, dehydration
6. Skin lesions
    (i) Pyoderma gangrenosum
    (ii) Aphthous ulcers
    (iii) Erythema nodosum
    (iv) Clubbing
7. Diffuse liver disease
8. Arthritis and uveitis
9. Amyloidosis after chronic abscesses
10. Carcinoma of colon

Ba enema
1. Loss of haustration
2. Straight, narrow, inelastic colon
3. May be 'spicules' due to tiny ulcer craters
4. May be filling defects due to 'pseudopolyps'

CIRRHOSIS

Cirrhosis is characterized by hepatic parenchymal damage with fibrosis and nodular regeneration throughout the liver, accompanied by distortion of the normal lobular pattern.

Causes of cirrhosis
1. Cryptogenic (idiopathic)
2. Alcoholism
3. Viral hepatitis (especially serum hepatitis)

4. 'Auto-immune' liver disease
   Primary biliary cirrhosis
   Active chronic hepatitis
5. Hepatotoxins, e.g. methotrexate, carbon tetrachloride

Clinical features of portal cirrhosis (Laennec)

(A) *Features of hepatic failure*
  (i) Firm hepatomegaly in the early stages
  (ii) Low grade fever
  (iii) Skin changes
      Jaundice in later stages
      'Spiders'
      Palmar erythema
      White nails
  (iv) Bleeding tendency (decreased coagulation factors)
  (v) Fatigue, weight loss, dyspepsia
  (vi) Foetor hepaticus
  (vii) Encephalopathy
      Lethargy
      Slow, slurred speech
      Flapping tremor
      Dementia
      Precoma progressing to delirium and coma
  (viii) Water retention
      Oedema
      Hyponatraemia

(B) *Features of portal hypertension*
  (i) Splenomegaly, often with pancytopenia (hypersplenism)
  (ii) GI bleeding from eosophageal varices
  (iii) Ascites (low plasma albumin is also necessary)

(C) *Other features*
  (i) Clubbing
  (ii) Hyperkinetic circulation
  (iii) Sexual changes
      Females: Erratic menstruation and breast atrophy
      Males: Gynaecomastia, testicular atrophy and scanty body hair
  (iv) Parotid enlargement ⎱
  (v) Dupuytren's contracture ⎰ in alcoholics
  (vi) Susceptibility to infections

Causes of cholestasis

1. Extra-hepatic
  (i)   Stone in common bile-duct (CBD)
  (ii) Carcinoma of head of pancreas or biliary tract
  (iii) Pressure on CBD from lymph nodes
  (iv) Stricture of CBD (post-operative or post-inflammatory)
  (v)   Developmental anomalies (rare)

2. Intra-hepatic
  (i)   Hepatitis
  (ii) Primary biliary cirrhosis
  (iii) Drugs — Hypersensitivity, e.g. chlorpromazine
                 Dose-related, e.g. methyltestosterone
  (iv) Pregnancy or oestrogen ingestion

JAUNDICE

Table 2. Summary of urinary and faecal bile pigment changes

	Obstructive	Hepatocellular failure with no obstruction	Haemolytic
Urinary Bilirubin	Increased	Normal or increased	Normal
Urinary Urobilinogen	Decreased	Normal or increased	Increased
Faecal Stercobilinogen	Decreased	Normal	Increased

GASTRO-INTESTINAL DISEASE AND DENTISTRY

1. Peptic ulceration and duodenal ulceration
It is said that these patients should have efficient masticatory ability to aid digestion. This is of doubtful significance.
Aspirin-containing analgesics should be avoided as they are irritant and tend to promote gastric bleeding.

2. Liver disease
Patients who have recently had jaundice may have an increased tendency to bleed due to reduced prothrombin synthesis.
Any patient with liver disease should be given drugs which are metabolised in the liver only with caution (e.g. tetracyclines).
Lignocaine hydrochloride and other amide local anaesthetics are metabolized in the liver. Thus dosages should be kept to the minimum.

Any patient who has had acute hepatitis within 6 weeks prior to consultation at a dentist could be Hepatitis B (Australia antigen) positive and should be barrier treated with appropriate precautions for urgent treatment and serological testing.

3. Intestinal disease
Coeliac disease and certain other gastro-intestinal disorders, e.g. Crohn's disease, may have gingival/mucosal manifestations. Coeliac disease associated with gluten enteropathy can rarely cause recurrent oral aphthous ulceration.

Renal system

FUNCTIONS OF THE KIDNEY

1. Maintenance of tissue fluids at constant composition.
2. Excretion of end-products of metabolism, e.g.
    urea from protein breakdown
    uric acid from breakdown of cell nuclei
    creatinine from muscle
3. Excretion of drugs and toxins
4. Secretion of erythropoietin, which stimulates red cell production in the marrow
5. Secretion of renin, which increases blood pressure and also stimulates aldosterone secretion by the adrenal cortex.

The kidneys excrete some substances (e.g. glucose) only when a certain concentration is exceeded in the blood. This threshold value varies for each substance. For glucose it is normally 10 mmol/litre (180 mg/100 ml) of blood, and glycosuria occurs only when this level is exceeded.

URINE

The kidneys receive approximately 25% of the cardiac output. The glomeruli filter off approximately 150 litres of fluid per day. Most of this is reabsorbed by the renal tubules. The daily urinary output is approximately 1.5 litres. This volume varies according to fluid intake and thus the specific gravity of urine varies. In severe renal disease the ability of the kidney to control the urinary output and its specific gravity is lost.

Causes of polyuria (increased urine production)

1. Excessive fluid intake (especially alcohol or coffee)
2. Chronic renal failure
3. Diabetes mellitus or diabetes insipidus
4. Diuretic drugs

68

Causes of oliguria (decreased urine production)
1. *Dehydration*
    (i) Decreased fluid intake
    (ii) Excessive sweating
    (iii) Diarrhoea, vomiting, gastric aspiration
2. *Reduced renal perfusion*
    (i) 'Shock'
    (ii) Cardiac failure
3. Acute renal failure

Protein
A trace of protein may be found in the urine of normal subjects, but marked proteinuria is always a sign of disease. Albumin is found most commonly, but in some rare diseases globulins occur in excess in the blood and leak into the urine.

Causes of proteinuria
1. *Contamination*
    In women, with vaginal secretion
    In men, with semen or prostatic secretion
2. *'Postural' (orthostatic) proteinuria*
    Disappears when the patient is horizontal, and is absent from the specimen passed on rising. It does not indicate disease.
3. *Renal disease*
    (i) Glomerulonephritis, especially in nephrotic syndrome
    (ii) Pyelonephritis
    (iii) Malignant hypertension
    (iv) Tuberculosis
4. *Disease of renal tract,* e.g. cystitis
5. *Slight albuminuria* often occurs in fevers or in congestive heart failure.
6. *Patients with multiple myeloma* secrete Bence-Jones protein, which coagulates on heating but redissolves on boiling.

Blood
Haematuria (red cells in urine) is distinguished from haemoglobinuria (Hb within urine) by microscopy.
Haemoglobinuria is a sign of haemolysis of red cells.

Causes of haematuria
1. *Kidney lesions*
    (i) Trauma
    (ii) Glomerulonephritis, pyelonephritis or TB
    (iii) Hypernephroma
2. *Renal tract lesions*
    (i) Cystitis or bladder tumour
    (ii) Calculi from kidney or bladder
    (iii) Prostatic disease, especially carcinoma
3. *Bleeding disease or anticoagulant overdose*

Sugars
The most important is glucose (glycosuria)

Causes of glycosuria
1. *Hyperglycaemic* (glucose over 10 mmol/litre blood)
2. *Low renal threshold* (defective tubular reabsorption)
   In this condition glucose leaks into the urine even though the blood sugar concentration is normal, and these patients are not diabetic. It is usually of no significance.
3. *Bile*
   Bile occurs in the urine when the patient is jaundiced, especially if this is due to biliary tract obstruction.
4. *Urobilin*
   This is formed in the intestine during the enterohepatic circulation of bile.
   Absence of urobilin from urine indicates complete biliary tract obstruction.
   Excess of urobilin is due to
   (i) Haemolysis (with excess bilirubin from Hb breakdown)
   (ii) Hepatic failure (inability of the liver to re-excrete urobilin)
5. *Ketones*
   The ketones (acetone and two more complex molecules) are derived from the excessive breakdown of fats. If they occur in the urine the patient is said to be ketotic.

Causes of ketosis
1. Starvation
2. Uncontrolled diabetes mellitus
3. Prolonged vomiting

RENAL FAILURE

This may be acute or chronic
In acute failure the kidneys may produce little urine (oliguria) or no urine (anuria). In chronic failure they may fail to respond to antidiuretic hormone leading to the constant production of large quantities of dilute urine of mixed specific gravity (usually 1.010). There may be abnormal urinary constituents, e.g. albumin, red cells, pus or casts. Casts are cylindrical fragments formed from protein in the lumen of the kidney tubules, and the presence of casts in the urine always indicates renal pathology.

Metabolic effects of renal failure
1. *Uraemia*
   Blood urea exceeding 5.5 mmol/litre (40 mg/100 ml); due to accumulation of protein metabolites
2. *Hyperkalaemia*
   Due to potassium retention

3. *Hyponatraemia*
   Due to loss of sodium in urine
4. *Hypoproteinamia*
   Due to loss of albumen
5. *Hypocalcaemia*
   Due to loss of calcium in urine
6. *Acidosis*
   (Decreased blood pH)

'URAEMIA'

This term is often used to refer to the overall clinical picture of advanced renal failure, rather than the accumulation of urea alone.

Clinical features of 'uraemia'
1. Loss of energy, drowsiness, confusion
2. Anorexia, nausea, vomiting, hiccups and occasionally ulcerative stomatitis
3. Pruritus, pallor and 'earthy' pigmentation
4. 'Air hunger' (Kussmaul breathing) due to acidosis
5. Cardiac arrhythmia or cardiac arrest, due to hyperkalaemia
6. Osteomalacia or secondary hyperparathyroidism, due to hypocalcaemia
In renal failure there may be an associated renin-induced hypertension, giving headaches, loss of vision, transient loss of consciousness or hemiplegia. These are strictly symptoms of the hypertension and not the uraemia. Such disturbance in cerebral function is called *hypertensive encephalopathy.*

Causes of uraemia
1. *Renal*
   Both kidneys must be extensively damaged.
   (i) Acute nephritis
   (ii) Chronic nephritis
   (iii) Chronic pyelonephritis
   (iv) Hypertensive renal disease
   (v) 'Crush syndrome'
   (vi) Analgesic nephropathy (due to paracetamol)
2. *Extra-renal*
   (i) Obstruction to urinary outlow e.g. prostatic enlargement
   (ii) Inadequate blood supply to kidney e.g. haemorrhage, shock
The distinction between the two types of uraemia is important as extra-renal causes are usually treatable and the uraemia is reversible, whilst renal causes are often irreversible.
Renal failure, other than for a short period, is lethal.

Treatment of 'uraemia'
This will vary according to whether the renal failure is acute or chronic.

ACUTE RENAL FAILURE

Causes
1. *'Shock'*
   (i) Blood loss or fluid loss
   (ii) Hypotension e.g. myocardial infarction
   (iii) Septicaemia
   (iv) Obstetric disasters e.g. abortion or ante-partum haemorrhage
2. *Acute glomerulonephritis or pyelonephritis*
3. *Severe crush injuries*

Treatment of acute renal failure
1. Correction of fluid and electrolyte loss. For an adult the fluid intake is about 500 ml plus the volume of urine passed in the previous 24 hours. It is usually given as a concentrated glucose solution to supply calories to minimize tissue breakdown.
2. An anabolic steriod to minimize tissue breakdown
3. Resonium A (binds potassium in the intestine) to lower plasma potassium
4. If necessary, peritoneal dialysis or haemodialysis
If recovery of renal function occurs the patient enters a diuretic phase, with large volumes of dilute urine. Large amounts of water, sodium and potassium are lost and may need to be replaced.

GLOMERULONEPHRITIS

This term is applied to diffuse inflammatory disease affecting the glomeruli. It is probably due to complex immunological reactions to a variety of antigenic stimuli, including infection with β-haemolytic streptococci or viruses. It is classified by the histological appearance of a renal biopsy specimen.
1. *Minimal change* — changes seen only on electron microscopy
2. *Membranous* — diffuse thickening of the glomerular capillary walls
3. *Proliferative* — increased number of cells in all glomeruli
4. *Focal* — proliferative changes seen in only some parts of some glomeruli
There are two main clinical types of glomerulonephritis:
1. Acute nephritis
2. Nephrotic syndrome
Either can develop hypertension or progress to chronic renal failure, and many intermediate types occur.

ACUTE NEPHRITIS

Clinical features
1. Often youngsters with a history of streptococcal tonsillitis one to three weeks previously
2. Sudden onset of headache, pyrexia, vomiting, loin pain
3. Scanty urine, with albuminuria and a smoky appearance due to haematuria
4. Moderate oedema, often periorbital, and worse in the morning

Prognosis
Most cases recover completely in a few weeks, but some die of acute renal failure or develop progressive chronic renal failure.

Treatment
1. Bed rest
2. Penicillin for a few days to eradicate streptococci
3. High calorie diet, with restriction of protein, fluid and salt until the diuretic phase occurs

NEPHROTIC SYNDROME

This is characterized by
1. Heavy proteinuria
2. Low plasma proteins
3. Massive oedema

Glomerulonephritis is by far the commonest cause of the nephrotic syndrome, but it is occasionally secondary to other disease, e.g. diabetes.

Clinical features
1. Insidious onset of oedema, with a pale puffy face. The oedema becomes generalized, often with ascites or pleural effusion.
2. Increased susceptibility to infections

Prognosis
Variable, but oedema may persist for months or years. Many patients ultimately develop renal failure.

Treatment
1. High protein diet with restriction of salt
2. Diuretics
3. Prednisone or immunosuppressive drugs such as azathioprine
4. Paracentesis (drainage) of ascites or pleural effusion

CHRONIC RENAL FAILURE

Common causes
1. Glomerulonephritis
2. Pyelonephritis   — bacterial
3. Malignant hypertension
4. Urinary tract obstruction e.g. stones or prostatic enlargement

Clinical features
1. *Nocturia* (increased nocturnal urine production) is an early symptom, followed eventually by polyuria
2. *'Uraemia'* develops insidiously

Treatment
1. Fluid intake should be at least 3 litres daily, because in chronic renal failure the excretion of urea etc, is proportional to the urinary flow. Salt supplements may be needed.
2. Low protein diet (e.g. 40 g daily). In more advanced cases the Giovanetti diet is used, with vitamin supplements.
3. Blood transfusion may be needed for severe anaemia
4. Hypertension should be controlled
5. Dialysis with artificial kidney or renal transplant should be considered

RENAL DIALYSIS

In this procedure the blood is artificially 'purified' in an extra-corporeal dialysis machine using semi-permeable membranes. 'Toxins' such as urea are thus removed from the blood, which is then returned to the patient's own circulation. The patient has an indwelling arterio-venous shunt in either arm or leg through which blood leaves and is returned. Dialysis has to be carried out twice each week for life or until kidney function adequately returns (or renal transplant is performed).
There are many problems associated with dialysis e.g.
1. Thrombosis of the arteriovenous shunt, which thus becomes defunct, and the number of available sites is limited
2. Deficiency of essential blood components e.g. calcium, which leads to osteomalacia, etc
3. Dialysis patients tend to develop rampant caries and periodontal disease. The reasons for this are not clear, but obviously such patients require careful dental care.

URINARY TRACT INFECTION

The urinary tract consists of the renal pelvis, ureter, bladder and urethra.

Cystitis

Inflammation of the bladder, usually due to bacterial infection. It predominantly affects women, since the short female urethra readily allows bacteria to spread from the perineum to the bladder. Infection can also descend from an infected kidney, and conversely infection of the lower urinary tract is often followed by acute pyelonephritis.

Other predisposing causes:
   (i) Retention of urine
  (ii) Calculi
 (iii) Bladder diverticula or cancer

Clinical features

1. Frequency of micturition, with dysuria
2. Cloudy urine with offensive odour
3. May be rigors, pyrexia and supra-pubic tenderness

ACUTE PYELONEPHRITIS

Infection of the renal pelvis, often also involving the kidney tissue.

Predisposing causes

1. Lower urinary tract infection, especially if accompanied by urinary stasis (e.g. pregnancy, prostatic hypertrophy, paraplegia etc)
2. Reflux of urine up the ureters due to urethral or ureteric dysfunction
3. Pre-existing renal disease
4. Pre-existing systemic disease e.g. diabetes mellitus

Clinical features

1. Sudden onset of fever, rigors and malaise
2. Pain and tenderness in one or both loins
3. Frequency, dysuria and cloudy offensive urine

Treatment of cystitis and acute pyelonephritis

1. High fluid intake
2. Antibacterial drugs according to bacterial sensitivity, e.g. sulphonamides, cotrimoxazole, ampicillin, nalidixic acid or nitrofurantoin
3. Sodium bicarbonate to keep the urine alkaline

Follow-up urine cultures are essential to ensure the infection is eradicated. The underlying cause should be treated if possible since recurrent infection can lead to fatal chronic pyelonephritis.

CHRONIC PYELONEPHRITIS

The pathogenesis is poorly understood, but recurrent infection seems to produce small scarred kidneys and eventual renal failure. In some cases the onset is insidious with sterile urine and no history of urinary tract infection.

Clinical features
1. May resemble acute pyelonephritis
2. Asymptomatic proteinuria for years, followed by progressive renal failure

Treatment
1. Prolonged treatment (several months) with appropriate anti-bacterial drugs according to sensitivity
2. Treatment of renal failure
   Renal failure is often precipitated by an exacerbation of the infection or an electrolyte disturbance (e.g. from prolonged vomiting).

CALCULI

Calculi (stones) may form either in the kidney or bladder, and they usually consist of calcium salts, phosphates, urates or mixtures. Factors which predispose to stone formation:
1. Excess calcium in the urine, e.g. hyperparathyroidism
2. Excess urates in the urine, e.g. gout
3. Urinary tract infection, e.g. cystitis
4. Statis of urine, e.g. prostatic enlargement

Clinical features
1. A stone may produce no symptoms if it remains in the kidney
2. A stone entering the ureter produces renal colic
In this condition there is paroxysmal severe pain in the loin radiating into the abdomen and groin, often with haematuria. The patient is often restless, sweating and vomiting.
3. A stone in the bladder may cause dysuria and frequency
4. Small stones may pass uneventfully through the urethra. Larger ones may lodge and cause retention of urine.

Nervous system

THE SENSORY SYSTEM

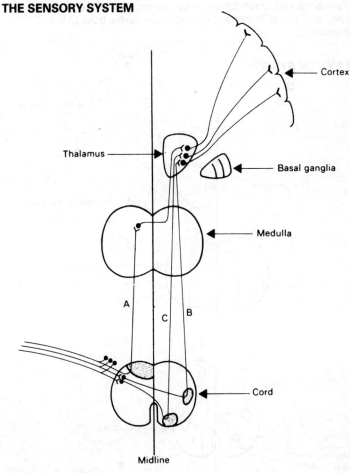

Fig. 3 The sensory system.
(Reproduced from Burton J L 1980 Aids to undergraduate medicine, 3rd edn, with permission.)

A. *Vibration, proprioception and ½ touch fibres* travel via posterior
   nerve roots up the posterior nerve roots up the posterior
   column without relaying in the cord. They relay in the medulla
   (nuclei gracilis and cuneatus) and cross the midline to continue
   as the medial lemniscus to the thalamus. Tertiary fibres travel
   via the posterior limb of the internal capsule to the sensory
   cortex (post-central gyrus).
B. *Pain and temperature fibres* relay in the cord, cross the midline
   immediately and travel in the *lateral* spinothalamic tract to the
   thalamus.
C. *Remainder of touch fibres* relay and cross the midline in the
   cord and travel in the *anterior* spinothalamic tract to the
   thalamus.

THE MOTOR SYSTEM

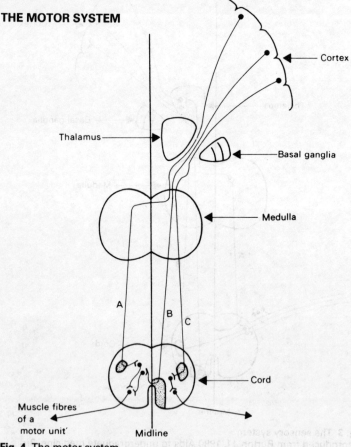

Fig. 4 The motor system.
(Reproduced from Burton J L 1980 Aids to Undergraduate medicine, 3rd
edn, with permission.)

Fibres pass downwards from the motor cortex (pre-central gyrus) into the posterior limb of the internal capsule. In the pons the fibres are scattered, but they regroup in the upper medulla to form protuberances called the pyramids.

A. In the lower medulla the majority of fibres decussate and descend in the *lateral* corticospinal (crossed pyramidal) tracts.

B. Some fibres do not decussate, but descend in the *anterior* cortico-spinal tract, and then cross in the anterior commissure of the cord.

C. A few fibres descend directly in the *lateral* corticospinal tract with the crossed fibres from the contralateral cortex.

Most fibres relay with internuncial cells in the cord, and the anterior horn cells and their fibres then form the 'final common pathway' to the motor end-plates in the muscle. The organization of movement is much more complex than this diagram suggests, since impulses are modified by the cerebellum, the extra-pyramidal system and proprioceptive and other sensations.

Signs of a lower motor neurone lesion
1. Weakness and wasting
2. Hypotonicity
3. Decreased reflexes
4. Fasciculation

Signs of an upper motor neurone lesion
1. Weakness
2. Spasticity
3. Increased tendon reflexes, with clonus
4. Extensor plantar response

CRANIAL NERVE SUPPLY
1. *Olfactory* Smell
2. *Optic* Vision
3. *Oculomotor*
   (i) *All ocular muscles, except superior oblique and lateral rectus*
   (ii) *Ciliary muscle*
   (iii) *Sphincter pupillae*
   (iv) *Levator palpebrae superioris*
4. *Trochlear* Superior oblique muscle
   N.B.Tested by asking patient to look down and *inwards*
5. *Trigeminal*
   (i) Sensory for face, cornea, sinuses, nasal mucosa, teeth, tympanic membrane and anterior two-thirds of tongue
   (ii) Motor to muscles of mastication
6. *Abducens* Lateral rectus muscle

   7. *Facial*
      (i) Motor to scalp and facial muscles of expression
      (ii) Taste in anterior two-thirds of tongue (via chorda tympani)
      (iii) Nerve to stapedius muscle
   8. *Auditory* Auditory and vestibular components
   9. *Glossopharyngeal*
      (i) Sensory for posterior one-third of tongue, pharynx and middle ear
      (ii) Taste fibres for posterior one-third of tongue
      (iii) Motor to middle ocnstrictor of pharynx and stylo-pharyngeus
   10. *Vagal*
      (i) Motor to soft palate, larynx and pharynx (from nucleus ambiguus)
      (ii) Sensory and motor for heart, respiratory passages and abdominal viscera (from dorsal nucleus)
   11. *Spinal accessory*
      (i) Motor to sterno-mastoid and trapezius
      (ii) Accessory fibres to vagus
   12. *Hypoglossal* Motor to tongue and hyoid bone depressors

Cervical sympathetic paralysis (Horner's)
   (i) Mild ptosis
   (ii) Enopthalmos
   (iii) Pupil constricted with no reaction to shading
   (iv) Reduced sweating on ipsilateral half of head and neck
   (v) Abolition of cilio-spinal reflex

Causes of Horner's syndrome
   (i) Carcinoma of apical bronchus
   (ii) Cervical sympathectomy
   (iii) Aortic aneurysm
   (iv) Syringobulbia or syringomyelia
   (v) Brachial plexus lesions (e.g. Klumpke's paralysis)

OPTIC PATHWAY

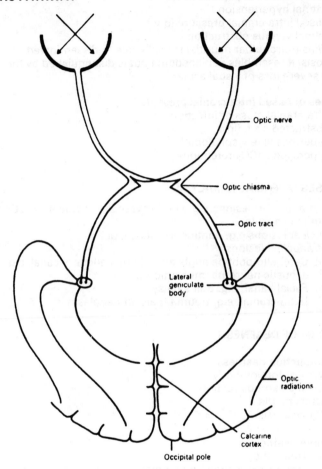

Fig. 5 Optic pathway.
(Reproduced from Burton J L 1980 Aids to undergraduate medicine, 3rd edn, with permission.)

PAPILLOEDEMA

Signs of papilloedema
1. Engorged retinal veins
2. Pink disc with blurred margin
3. Loss of 'cupping'
4. Cribrosa not visible
5. Flame-shaped haemorrhages

Common causes of papilloedema
1. Arterial hypertension
2. Raised intra-cranial pressure (q.v.)
3. Retinal venous obstruction

Papillitis (retrobulbar neuritis) is usally due to disseminated sclerosis. It resembles papilloedema but is distinguished by the early severe loss of visual acuity.

Causes of raised intra-cranial pressure
1. Intra-cranial mass or infection
2. Obstructed c.s.f. flow
3. Hypertensive encephalopathy
4. Hypercapnia (CO_2 retention)

CAUSES OF FACIAL PARALYSIS

1. *Supra-nuclear* lesions e.g. cerebrovascular accident affecting internal capsule
2. *Nuclear* lesions e.g. pontine neoplasm, polio
3. *Infranuclear* lesions
   (i) Cerebello-pontine angle and internal auditory canal, e.g. acoustic neuroma, meningioma
   (ii) Facial canal, e.g. Bell's palsy
   (iii) Extra-cranial, e.g. trauma, parotid neoplasm

CAUSES OF DEAFNESS

1. **Conduction deafness**
   (i) Wax or foreign-body
   (ii) Eustachian obstruction
   (iii) Otitis media
   (iv) Otosclerosis

2. **Nerve deafness**
   (i) Traumatic
      Chronic exposure to loud noise
      Fractures of petrous temporal bone
   (ii) Infective
      Congenital syphilis
      Rubella syndrome
      Mumps, influenza
   (iii) Toxic
      Aspirin, quinine
      Antibiotics, e.g. streptomycin, neomycin
   (iv) Degenerative
      Presbyacusis

Rinne's test
The ability to hear a tuning fork through air and through the mastoid process are compared. In *normal* people and in *nerve* deafness the air-conducted sound is louder, whereas in conduction deafness it is softer.

Weber's test
The base of the fork is placed on the centre of the forehead: in *nerve* deafness the note is heard in the *normal* ear, whereas in conduction deafness it is heard in the deaf ear.

COMMON INTRACRANIAL NEOPLASMS

Children
Medulloblastoma
Astrocytoma

Adults
Glioma
Meningioma
Metastatic cancer
Acoustic neuroma
Pituitary tumour

Clinical features of intracranial neoplasm
1. Raised intra-cranial pressure
     (i) Headache, worse on straining and on waking
    (ii) Drowsiness
   (iii) Bradycardia
    (iv) Vomiting
     (v) Papilloedema
2. Progressive loss of neurological function or focal neurological signs (q.v.)
3. Epilepsy
4. Mental symptoms, e.g. personality change, apathy, dementia

Localization of cortical lesions by focal neurological signs

Frontal
1. Mental disturbance
   dementia
   apathy
   inappropriate emotion
2. Epilepsy
3. Grasp reflex
4. Unilateral anosmia

Pre-central
1. Jacksonian epilepsy
2. Contralateral spastic hemiplegia

Parietal
1. Sensory disturbance, e.g. lack of two point discrimination
2. Visual aphasia
3. Homonymous hemianopia
4. Apraxia
5. Astereognosis

Temporal
1. Anterior lesions — motor aphasia
2. Posterior lesions — auditory aphasia
2. Homonymous hemianopia or quadrantanopia
3. Psychomotor epilepsy

Occipital
Visual field defects

Signs of a cerebellar lesion
1. Intention tremor
2. 'Scanning' speech
3. Nystagmus worse on looking to the side of the lesion
4. Limb ataxia with characteristic gait
5. Hypotonia and pendular reflexes

Causes of a cerebellar lesion
1. Disseminated sclerosis
2. Neoplasms
    (i) In the cerebellum, e.g. medulloblastoma
    (ii) Neuropathy secondary to malignancy such as bronchial
        carcinoma
3. Cerebellar abscess (often secondary to otitis media)
4. Vertebro — basilar insufficiency
5. Idopathic degeneration, e.g. primary cerebellar atrophy
6. Rare hereditary and familial ataxias, e.g. Friedreich's

SUBARACHNOID HAEMORRHAGE

Common causes
1. Ruptured 'berry' aneurysm (85%)
2. Cerebral angioma (10%)

Clinical features
1. Often occurs in middle life
2. Sudden onset of catastrophic headache, usually occipital. Often precipitated by straining
3. Small leakages — delirium or confusion but no loss of consciousness
   Bigger bleeds — vomiting, convulsions and coma
4. Meningism
5. Plantar responses are usually extensor
6. May be slow pulse, or hypertension
7. Occasionally squint, papilloedema, retinal haemorrhage and small sluggish pupils
8. May be pain in back due to blood in spinal theca

CHRONIC SUBDURAL HAEMATOMA

Cause
Rupture of cortical veins as they cross the subdural space. May be traumatic or spontaneous.

Clinical features
1. Often elderly patients, after a trivial head injury
2. Latent period of days or months occurs before symptoms develop
3. Gradual onset of headaches, memory loss, dementia, confusion, drowsiness and eventual coma. Symptoms fluctuate from day to day, with lucid intervals.
4. May be signs of an intra-cranial space-occupying lesion, with localizing signs

EXTRA–DURAL HAEMATOMA

Cause
1. Any age, but often young adults with scalp oedema above the ear
2. Concussion may be followed by recovery of consciousness for minutes or hours before the onset of drowsiness and deepening coma
3. Signs of intra-cranial compression
4. Ipsilateral 3rd nerve palsy due to cerebral herniation
5. Progressive contralateral hemiplegia
The signs develop rapidly·and immediate operation to relieve the pressure is mandatory.

CAUSES OF CEREBRAL INFARCTION
1. Atheroma of intra- or extra-cranial arteries
2. Cerebral emboli
   (i) atrial fibrillation
   (ii) myocardial infarct
   (iii) bacterial endocarditis
3. Cerebral ischaemia due to severe hypotension
4. Cerebral arterial spasm, e.g. migraine or following subarachnoid haemorrhage
5. Hypoxia, e.g.
   cardiac arrest
   carbon monoxide poisoning
   pulmonary emboli

CAUSES OF COMA
1. Syncope (q.v.)
2. Head injury
3. Epilepsy
4. Drugs or toxins (especially alcohol)
5. CVA (thrombosis, embolism or haemorrhage)
6. Raised intra-cranial pressure
7. Metabolic
   (i) Hypoglycaemia
   (ii) Diabetic ketoacidaemia
   (iii) Hepatic, renal or adrenal failure
   (iv) Myxoedema
   (v) Electrolyte imbalance
8. Acute CNS infection, e.g. meningitis, encephalitis
9. Acute systemic infection, e.g. septicaemia
10. Hysteria, hypnosis
11. Hypo- or hyperthermia

SYNCOPE

A transient loss of consciousness caused by cerebral anoxia, usually due to inadequate blood flow.

Causes
1. Vasovagal
   (i) Emotion, heat or standing still
   (ii) Loss of blood or plasma
   (iii) Postural hypotension, e.g. drugs or prolonged recumbency
2. Cardiac
   (i) Stokes-Adams (heart block)
   (ii) Ventricular tachycardia or fibrillation
   (iii) Aortic stenosis

3. Arterial occlusion
   (i) Atheroma or embolism (carotid or vertebro-basilar)
   (ii) Cervical spondylosis
   (iii) Strangulation
4. Anoxaemia
   (i) High altitude
   (ii) Anaemia

ABNORMAL GAITS

N.B. Most cases are due to lesions of bone, joint or skin.

'Neurological' gaits
1. *Upper motor neurone hemiplegia*
   Arm adducted and internally rotated
   Elbow flexed and pronated
   Fingers flexed
   Foot plantar-flexed, with leg swung in a lateral arc
2. *Spasti paraplegia*
   Stiff jerky 'scissors' gait, with complicated assisting movements
   of upper limbs
3. *Parkinsonism*
   Small shuffling hurried steps
   Flexion of neck, elbows, wrists and MP joints with thumbs
   adducted
4. *Cerebellar lesion*
   'Drunken' gait on a broad base. Feet raised excessively and
   placed carefully, with patient looking ahead. Tends to fall to side
   of lesion.
5. *Posterior column lesion*
   Patient walks on a broad base but bangs feet down clumsily and
   tends to look at feet. Rombergism is present.
6. *High-stepping gait*
   Due to foot drop
7. *Proximal myopathy*
   Waddling gait with broad base, lordosis and marked body
   swing. This gait occurs also in congenital hip dislocation and
   pregnancy.
8. *Hysterical*
   Usually bizarre and inconsistent, and the patient rarely falls
9. *Involuntary movements*
   (i) *Choreiform* — Jerky movements of short duration, affecting
      limbs and face
   (ii) *Athetoid* — slow writhing of arms and legs with flexed
      fingers, thumb and wrist

CLASSIFICATION OF SPEECH DEFECTS

1. Dysphasia (disorder in use of symbols for communication whether spoken, heard, written or read)
2. Dysarthria (disorder of articulation)
3. Dysphonia (disorder of vocalization)
4. Dementia (intellectual deterioration)

Causes of dysphasia

 (i) Motor — due to lesion of inferior frontal gyrus of dominant frontal lobe (Broca's area)
(ii) Sensory — due to lesion of dominant temporo-parietal cortex

Causes of dysarthria

1. Bulbar or pseudo-bulbar palsy
2. Basal ganglia lesions
3. Cerebellar lesions
4. Weakness or paralysis of facial muscles
5. Oral lesions including denture problems

Causes of dysphonia

1. Functional (hysteria)
2. Lesions of recurrent laryngeal nerve
3. Vocal cord lesion (infection, tumour, etc)

SYRINGOMYELIA AND SYRINGOBULBIA

Syringomyelia

Usually starts in base of posterior horn of cervical region

Clinical features
Insidious onset of
1. Weakness and wasting of small muscles of hand
2. Sensory loss in hand (pain and temperature only)
3. Trophic changes
     (i) Cyanosis of fingers
    (ii) Ulceration and scarring
   (iii) Swollen fingers due to subcutaneous hypertrophy
4. Loss of tendon reflexes
5. Painful arm
6. Spastic paraplegia
7. Charcot joints (neck and shoulders)

Syringobulbia

Medulla may be initial site, or may be involved by upward extension from cord.

Clinical features
1. Facial pain or sensory loss (Cr. 5)
2. Vertigo and nystagmus (Cr. 8)
3. Facial, palatal or laryngeal palsy (Cr. 7, 9, 10, 11)
4. Wasted tongue (Cr. 12)
5. Horner's syndrome (Sympathetic)

BULBAR PALSY
Bilateral *lower* motor neurone lesions of the bulbar nuclei (9, 10, 11 and 12 with lowermost part of 7).

Clinical features
1. Dysarthria
2. Dysphagia, especially with fluids
3. Wasted fibrillating tongue
4. Palatal paralysis

Causes
1. Motor neurone disease
2. Polio
3. Encephalitis
4. Syringobulbia

PSEUDO-BULBAR PALSY

Bilateral *upper* motor neurone lesions of the same nuclei

Clinical features
1. Dysarthria
2. Dysphagia
3. Spastic tongue
4. Exggerated jaw-jerk (spastic masseters)
5. Emotional lability

Causes
1. Ischaemia of internal capsule
2. Motor neurone disease
3. Disseminated sclerosis

PERIPHERAL NEUROPATHY

Characterized by symmetrical flaccid weakness and sensory changes of 'glove and stocking' distribution.

Causes of polyneuropathy
1. *Many cases are idiopathic*
2. *Drugs and chemicals*
    Isoniazid
    Lead, mercury
    Many organic chemicals
3. *Metabolic*
    Diabetes mellitus
    Amyloidosis
    Acute intermittent porphyria
4. *Deficiency states*
    B_{12} deficiency
    Alcoholism
    Beri-beri
    Pellagra
5. *Infections*
    Leprosy
    Diphtheria
    Tetanus
    Botulism
6. *Miscellaneous*
    'Acute infective polyneuritis' of Guillain-Barré
    Collagen-vascular disease, esp. polyarteritis and rheumatoid
    disease
    Malignancy
    Sarcoidosis
7. *Congenital*
    Rate hereditary ataxias and neuropathies

DISSEMINATED SCLEROSIS

Characterized by multiple CNS lesions scattered in time and place.

Clinical features
1. Spastic weakness, usually starting in legs
2. Retrobulbar neuritis
    Misty vision
    Painful eye movements
    Slightly swollen optic disc
    Central scotoma
3. Numbness and paraesthesia
4. Diplopia
5. Vertiga
6. Cerebellar signs
    Intention tremor
    Nystagmus
    'Scanning' speech

7. Sphincter disturbance and impotence
8. Euphoria or other mental change
9. Painful flexor spasms

CAUSES OF EPILEPSY

1. **Idopathic**

2. **Focal cerebral lesions**
  (i) Birth injury or cerbral malformation
  (ii) Tumour
  (iii) Trauma, scar, irradiation atrophy
  (iv) Vascular
    CVA
    Hypertension
  (v) Infection
    Encephalitis or meningitis
    Abscess or tuberculoma
    Syphilis (GPI or gumma)
  (vi) Degenerative disease, e.g. presenile dementia

3. **Metabolic**
  (i) Pyrexia in children
  (ii) Anoxia, hypoglycaemia or hypocalcaemia
  (iii) Electrolyte imbalance, e.g. water intoxication
  (vi) Uraemia
  (v) Hepatic coma
  (vi) Drugs and toxins
    Lead poisoning
    Withdrawal of alcohol or barbiturates

HEADACHE

The brain itself is insensitive to pain, but the vessels and meninges are innervated with pain receptors and fibres. Tension on these structures causes headache.

Causes of Headache
1. *Psychogenic* — pain with no organic cause. Often stress related.
2. *Vascular*
    (i) Migraine
      Often familial and may occur as a reaction to stress. Attack often starts as a visual aura, with a blind spot and saw-toothed flashing 'lights' (fortification spectrum). Severe unilateral headache follows. The *aura* is thought to represent vascular constriction, which is followed by severe vasodilatation giving the headache. The patient may have

transient weakness or loss of sensation, as well as
photophobia and nausea.
Ergotamine may be used to treat the attacks.
 (ii) Hypertension
Headache is a common presenting symptom of this
condition. The mechanism is uncertain.
(iii) Sub-arachnoid haemorrhage
(iv) Space-occupying tumour
 (v) Temporal arteritis, due to inflammation of unknown
aetiology of the temporal arteries. Diagnosis is by biopsy of
the artery. The temporalis muscles in this condition may
show a type of intermittent claudication during mastication.
Visual disturbances occur too, which may lead to blindness.
3. *Infections*
 (i) General e.g. influenza, typhoid
 (ii) Local e.g. Sinusitis (especially frontal, meningitis,
encephalitis
4. *Referred pain*
E.g. glaucoma, 'eye-strain' or sinusitis

Neurology and the dental surgeon
1. Cranial nerve lesions
e.g. Trigeminal neuralgia
Herpes zoster
Facial nerve paralysis (upper and lower motor neurone
paralysis)
2. Loss of consciousness
Careful diagnosis is necessary.
A simple fainting attack (vaso-vagal syncope) must be
distinguished from epilepsy, myocardial infarct, Stokes-Adams
attack, and 'stroke' due to cerebro-vascular accident
3. Disseminated sclerosis may have as its early sign pain similar to
that seen in trigeminal neuralgia
4. Patients who have had a cerebro-vascular accident must not be
given a general anaesthetic in a dental surgery

Rheumatology

Patterns of polyarthropathy

Primary osteoarthrosis
Symmetrical, affecting many joints
1. Knees
2. Great toes and thumbs: MP joints
3. Fingers: terminal IP joints
4. Acromio-clavicular joints
5. Small joints of spine

Secondary osteoarthrosis
Asymmetrical, affecting weight-bearing joints
1. Knee
2. Hip
3. Intervertebral discs

Rheumatoid arthritis
1. Hands: intercarpal joints, MP joints and proximal IP joints
2. Feet: tarsal and lateral MP joints
3. Knees
4. Small joints of cervical spine and subacromial bursae

Ankylosing spondylitis
1. Spine and both sacro-iliac joints
2. Knees, shoulders, wrists

Psoriasis
1. Hands, terminal IP joints
2. Sacro-iliac joints
3. 'Rheumatoid' pattern

Reiter's
1. Ankles and all joints of feet
2. Knees
3. Hips, sacro-iliac joint and spine

Causes of a single hot red joint
1. Traumatic, e.g. sprained ankle
2. Septic arthritis
3. May be secondary to penetrating injury, osteomyelitis, septicaemia, rheumatoid arthritis or osteoarthrosis.
3. Gout or pseudo-gout (chondrocalcinosis or periarticular calcification)
4. Haemophilia
5. Gonococcal arthritis
6. Occasionally rheumatoid arthritis

Causes of a transient 'flitting' arthritis
1. Rheumatic fever
2. Henoch–Schönlein purpura
3. Serum sickness and drug reactions
4. SLE
5. Systemic infections eg. bacterial endocarditis, rubella
6. Reiter's disease

Clinical features of polyarteritis nodosa
Usually young or middle-aged men
1. Fever, malaise, weight-loss
2. Gastro-intestinal ischaemia
   central abdominal pain
   bleeding
3. Proteinuria and haematuria. Hypertension is common
4. Peripheral neuropathy, often painful
   Focal CNS lesions
5. Arthralgia and myalgia
6. Myocardial ischaemia
7. Skin lesions
   nodules
   livedo reticularis
   necrosis and ulceration

Clinical features of systemic lupus erythematosus
Usually young or middle-aged women
1. Fever, malaise, weight-loss
2. Arthralgia, flitting or episodic
3. Skin changes
   (i) Rash, classically in butterly distribution. May be erythematous, urticated or purpuric
   (ii) Alopecia
   (iii) Dilated nail fold capillaries
   (iv) Raynaud's phenomenon
4. Proteinuria, glomerulonephritis, nephrotic syndrome or hypertension

5. Lymphadenopathy
6. Myocarditis, endocarditis (Libman–Sacks), or pericarditis
7. Pleurisy with effusion, pneumonitis
8. Hepatomegaly and splenomegaly
9. Pancytopenia. May be haemolysis.
10. Psychosis, neuropathy, or epilepsy. May be retinal exudates.
11. Gastrointestinal upsets (nausea, pain, diarrhoea, etc)

Dermatology

ECZEMA

Eczema is a distinctive inflammatory response of the skin, characterized histologically by spongiosis (epidermal oedema) and clinically by clustered papulo-vesicles with erythema and scaling. Many cases have a multifactorial aetiology.

Types of eczema

Exogenous
1. Primary irritant dermatitis, e.g. due to caustics, detergents or solvents
2. Allergic contact dermatitis, e.g. due to hypersensitivity to metals, rubber, medicaments, etc
3. Infective dermatitis, e.g. around infected wounds or ulcers

Endogenous
1. Atopic dermatitis (infantile eczema)
2. Seborrhoeic dermatitis
3. Discoid eczema
4. Pompholyx — vesicles on palms or soles
5. Pityriasis alba — patches of scaly eczema which leave depigmented areas
6. Asteatotic aczema — due to excessive drying ('chapping')
7. Gravitational eczema — secondary to venous insufficiency

PSORIASIS

Distinctive morphological types
1. Nummular — discoid plaques, which may be confluent
2. Guttate — 'showers' of small lesions, often post-streptococcal
3. Erythrodermic — very widespread erythema, with exfoliation
4. Generalized pustular psoriasis
5. Pustular eruptions of the hands and feet
Napkin psoriasis' (psoriasiform lesions in infants) may be related to *Candida* infection.

BLISTERING ERUPTIONS

Common
1. Viral
    Herpes simplex
    Herpes zoster — varicella
2. Impetigo
3. Insect bites
4. Bullous eczema and pompholyx
5. Drugs, e.g. photosensitivity due to nalidixic acid

Uncommon
6. Erythema multiforme ⎤
7. Dermatitis herpetiformis ⎟ sub-epidermal
8. Pemphigoid ⎟
9. Porphyria cutanea tarda ⎦
10. Pemphigus group   Intra-epidermal

Causes of leg ulcers
1. Venous stasis
2. Ischaemia
    Atheroma
    Arteritis
3. Neuropathy
    Diabetes mellitus
    Spina bifida
    Leprosy (in endemic areas)
4. Rheumatoid arthritis — ulceration is multifactorial
5. Malignancy — usually squamous-cell skin carcinoma
6. Pyoderma gangrenosum — often due to ulcerative colitis
Many leg ulcers have a multifactorial aertiology, e.g. ischaemia, anaemia, stasis and infection.

Causes of alopecia
1. Male-pattern baldness
2. Idiopathic diffuse alopecia of women — usually
    post-menopausal
3. 'Telogen effluvium' — loss of club hairs after febrile illness,
    surgery or parturition
4. Alopecia areata
5. Drugs
    Cytotoxic agents
    Anticoagulants
6. Scalp infection
    Fungi
    Pyogenic bacteria

7. Systemic disease
   Hypothyroidism
   Fe deficiency
8. Traumatic
   Scalping injury or burns
   Traction from rollers
   Excessive bleaching, perming, etc
9. Dermatoses
   Psoriasis
   Discoid lupus erythematosus
   Lichen planus
10. Congenital — rare

Causes of diffuse hyperpigmentation

1. *Congenital*
   (i) Racial or genetic
2. *Physical agents*
   (i) Radiation, e.g. UVR
   (ii) Chronic rubbing, e.g. 'vagabond's itch'
3. *Post-inflammatory*, e.g. erythroderma
4. *Endocrine* (Excess ACTH, MSH or oestrogen)
   (i) Pregnancy, oral contraceptives
   (ii) Hypoadrenalism
   (iii) Acromegaly
   (iv) ACTH therapy or ectopic ACTH from carcinoma
5. *Metabolic*
   (i) Cachexia
   (ii) Uraemia
   (iii) Hepatic disease, especially biliary cirrhosis
   (iv) Haemochromatosis
   (v) Malabsorption
6. *Drugs and Chemicals*
   (i) Arsenicals
   (ii) Busulphan
   (iii) Chlorpromazine
   (iv) Photodynamic agents, e.g. psoralens
7. *Pigmentation not due to melanin*
   (i) Jaundice — yellow
   (ii) Carotenaemia — yellow
   (iii) Mepacrine — yellow
   (iv) Argyria — grey

Causes of erythema nodosum

1. Sarcoidosis
2. Streptococcal infection
3. TB
4. Sulphonamides
5. Ulcerative colitis or Crohn's disease

6. Other infections, e.g.
   Leprosy
   Systemic mycoses
   Toxoplasmosis

Oral ulcerative lesions

1. Infective
(a) Herpes simplex
(b) Herpes zoster
(c) Hand-foot-mouth disease
(d) Herpangina
(e) Chicken pox (varicella)
(f) Candidosis
(g) Syphilis (primary, secondary or tertiary)

2. Immunologically based
(a) Recurrent oral ulceration (aphthae, major and minor; herpetiform)
(b) Behçet's syndrome
(c) Lichen planus
(d) Pemphigus vulgaris
(e) Mucous membrane pemphigoid
(f) Erythema multiforme
(g) Lupus erythematosus

Factors which predispose to oral candidosis
1. Trauma, eg. ill-fitting dentures
2. Serious illness eg. cancer or untreated diabetes mellitus
3. Broad spectrum antibiotics
4. Systemic steroids or immunosuppressive drugs
5. Iron deficiency

Skin tumours

Malignant
1. Basal cell carcinoma (rodent ulcer)
2. Squamous carcinoma
3. Malignant melanoma
4. Metastases or lymphoma

Benign
1. Melanocytic naevus ('mole')
2. Basal cell papilloma ('seborrhoeic wart')
3. Squamous papilloma
4. Kerato-acanthoma
5. Haemangioma
6. Pyogenic granuloma
7. Dermatofibroma (histiocytoma)
8. Epidermoid cyst ('wen')

Management of medical emergencies

CARDIAC ARREST

Immediately call the 'cardiac arrest team' and give a sharp thump on the praecordium. Clear the airway, start artificial respiration (mouth-to-mouth or Ambu bag) and external cardiac compression. If the bed is sprung, move the patient to the floor.

When help arrives they will arrange intubation and artificial ventilation with oxygen, and obtain an ECG.

Acid-base balance must be corrected under laboratory control, and mannitol infusion may be required for cerebral oedema.

MASSIVE PULMONARY EMBOLISM

Resuscitate the patient with external cardiac compression, oxygen administration. Vasopressor drugs and correction of acidosis requires expert advice.

Some advocate a large dose of heparin (15 000 units i.v.) to block serotonin release from the thrombus.

Subsequently therapy depends on the severity of the condition
  (i) Patients likely to die within an hour or so — bypass embolectomy (if facilities available)
 (ii) Slightly less critically ill patients — streptokinase infusion
(iii) Milder cases — heparin followed by oral anticoagulants

ACUTE ANAPHYLAXIS

The 'shock' is due to:
 (i) respiratory obstruction (laryngeal oedema and severe bronchospasm)
(ii) circulatory collapse (low plasma volume due to leakage of fluid into interstitial tissues)

In anaphylaxis due to an injection or sting, apply a tourniquet to the injected part if possible. For dental injections this is not possible. Hydrocortisone 300 mg i.v. should be given immediately together with 0.5 ml adrenaline (1:1000) subcutaneously. The adrenaline should *not* be repeated, as it may accumulate at the injection site

and be absorbed rapidly when the circulation improves. Some authors also advocate an antihistamine, e.g. promethazine 50 mg i.v.
Resuscitation with external cardiac compression, intubation (or tracheostomy) and mechanical ventilation may be required. Restoration of plasma volume by infusion of fluid is necessary.

DIABETIC HYPOGLYCAEMIC COMA

This can occur in the dental chair in poorly controlled or unstable diabetics as a result of fear, infection or inability to eat due to dental sepsis/pain, especially when there has been no adjustment of the insulin dosage. Signs are of visual disturbance, aggression, hunger-pains, pallor, sweating and unconciousness. Treatment is to give glucose by mouth or 20–50 ml 50% dextrose i.v.

DIABETIC KETOACIDAEMIC COMA

No inflexible rules can be given, since individual patients vary in their requirements. Treatment must be monitored throughout by frequent biochemical and clinical monitoring by experts. In the dental chair this is a most unlikely event. The hospital management of such a coma is along the following lines:
1. Treat the precipitating cause, e.g. infection
2. Blood analysis for glucose, urea and electrolytes, haematocrit and arterial blood pH
3. 40 to 120 units of soluble insulin ½ i.v. and ½ i.m. is given. The dose depends on whether the patient is a new diabetic or not, the degree of dehydration and shock, the presence or absence of infection, the depth of coma and the pre-coma daily insulin requirement.
4. Physiological saline infusion — 2 litres in the first 2 hours, then 1 litre every 2 hours. In old people or those with cardiac disease this may precipitate cardiac failure.
5. Potassium 20 mmol/h may be added to the infusion after the first hour
6. If initial pH is 7.00 or below, 100 mmol sodium bicarbonate i.v. is given and plasma sodium and bicarbonate repeated
7. Blood glucose, urea and electrolytes checked after 1 hour following the first dose of insulin, and 2-hourly thereafter. If the first post-insulin blcod glucose is *higher* than the initial glucose, *double* the initial dose of insulin is given. Soluble insulin is given 2-hourly thereafter in a dose depending on the rate of fall of blood glucose.
8. When blood glycose reaches 16 mmol/l, the saline infusion is replaced with 5% dextrose and insulin added by a 'sliding scale' according to urine glucose

'STATUS EPILEPTICUS'

Establish an adequate airway and give oxygen
Give 2 to 15 mg diazepam (Valium) by slow i.v. injection until
convulsions cease. Set up intravenous infusion of diazepam. Adjust
dose to prevent convulsions but beware of respiratory depression.
If venepuncture is impossible give 10 mg i.m. A suitable alternative
is paraldehyde (5 ml into each of 2 i.m. sites). Failure to control
seizures is an indication for curarization and ventilation. Seek
expert advice.

'STATUS ASTHMATICUS'

Administer oxygen with a Ventimask (35%)
Give aminophylline 250 to 500 mg by slow i.v. injection and
hydrocortisone 300 mg i.v. followed by a further 200 mg every 2
hours if necessary. Never sedate. Refer patient for further care to
hospital.

MANAGEMENT OF ACUTE POISONING

General principles and medical management

1. Prevent further absorption
Stomach washout is advisable except in the following
circumstances:
   (i) Corrosive and oil-based poisons
  (ii) Drowsy or comatose patients (unless a cuffed endotracheal
       tube is used)
 (iii) Delay of 4 h or more after ingestion (except after salicylates or
       tricyclics, in which stomach emptying is delayed)
Emetics should not be used

2. Intensive supportive treatment
   (i) Nurse prone and clear the airways
  (ii) Use artificial ventilation if minute volume is less than 4 litres
 (iii) Maintain hydration
  (iv) Treat hyper- or hypothermia
   (v) Monitor heart rate, blood pressure, peripheral perfusion and
       urine output
  (vi) Treat convulsions and arrhythmias

3. Antidotes and elimination of poison
   (i) Forced alkaline diuresis for weak acids, e.g. salicylates
  (ii) Dialysis is rarely useful, since most drugs do not dialyse freely
 (iii) Specific antidotes, e.g. naloxone for morphine

Barbiturates
Intensive supportive treatment.
Forced diuresis should be considered for phenobarbitone.

Salicylates
Absorption is slow, therefore stomach washout is advisable.
Expect complicated metabolic disturbances, e.g. respiratory alkalosis, metabolic acidosis and hypoprothrombinaemia.
Forced alkaline diuresis is very effective, but dangerous in elderly and in cardiac or renal failure or if not properly monitored.
Blood salicylate level is a good guide to severity of poisoning.

Ethanol
Prevention of aspiration of vomitus is important.
In severe cases gastric lavage is needed, with supportive therapy as required (artificial ventilation, etc).
In very severe poisoning peritoneal dialysis or haemodialysis is indicated.

Iron salts
High mortality in children if untreated. Symptoms are GI irritation, dehydration and delayed damage to liver and CNS.
Empty the stomach immediately by inducing vomiting and follow with gastric lavage using desferrioxamine solution (2 g in 1 litre).
Leave 10 g desferrioxamine in 50 ml water in the stomach and give 2 g of desferrioxamine i.m.

Carbon monoxide
Remove the patient from the poisonous atmosphere, clear the airway and give artificial respiration with 100% oxygen with the patient prone.
After spontaneous breathing starts there may be relapse into coma due to cerebral oedema, which may require i.v. infusion of 500 ml of 20 per cent mannitol.
Anoxic heart or brain damage may occur.

Narcotics (morphine, etc.)
Hypoventilation should be treated with naloxone 0.4 mg i.v. which acts within 2 min and may be repeated at 3 min intervals.

Phenothiazines
Little disturbance of consciousness and respiratory depression, but drugs for convulsions and cardiac arrhythmias may be needed.

Tricyclic antidepressives

These cause dry mouth, dilated pupils, disturbed consciousness, cardiac arrhythmias and in severe cases respiratory failure and hypotension. ECG monitoring is advisable. Physostigmine 1–3 mg i.v. over 2 min will reverse CNS effects and will counteract some cardiac effects.

Drug interactions with dental local anaesthetics containing adrenaline will produce a hypertensive crisis which should be controlled by phentolamine mesylate (Rogitine) 5 mg i.v. *slowly* until condition improves.

Petroleum products and paraffin (kerosene)

Gastric lavage is contraindicated because aspiration of a small amount causes pneumonitis. Absorption from the stomach is slowed by giving 250 ml of liquid paraffin.

Cyanide

Speed is essential. Inject two 20 ml ampoules of 1.5% dicobalt tetracemate (Kelocyanor) intravenously, followed by 20 ml of 50% glucose.

This treatment is replacing the previously recommended regime of breaking an ampoule of amyl nitrite under the patient's nose and then injecting sodium nitrite and sodium thiosulphate intravenously.

Gastric lavage and artifical ventilation with oxygen are also recommended.

Paracetamol

A toxic metabolite causes hepatic damage within 4 days. Oral methionine or i.v. cysteamine may prevent this damage if given within 10 h of ingestion.

Index